Inner Cycles of Health

LIVING WITH MS

Inner Cycles of Health

Living With MS

Marilyne V. Moyers-Mabery

Writers Club Press
San Jose New York Lincoln Shanghai

Inner Cycles of Health
Living With MS

Writers Club Press
an imprint of iUniverse, Inc.

For information address:
iUniverse, Inc.
5220 S. 16th St., Suite 200
Lincoln, NE 68512
www.iuniverse.com

ISBN: 0-595-20840-1

To my friends and family who have encouraged me
by teaching me how to accept their love and help knowing
I rightly deserve the blessing of their caring concern.

COURAGE AND TENACITY ARE STRANGE BEDFELLOWS THAT
TEACH LESSONS THAT ARE UNENDING.

M. V. MOYERS-MABERY 4/94

CONTENTS

FOREWORD

MY MILLENNIUM PLEDGE TO YOU MY READERS

The riveting moment of my life was getting the positive diagnoses, in 1978, of having Multiple Sclerosis. At the time I was a medical student, a new wife, and working the summer as a park ranger in one of the most beautiful places in North America, Canyonlands National Park, in southern Utah.

The mystery complaints I had baffled physicians with for the past five years now had a name, MS, this elated me. It gave purpose to my life. The challenge soon grew into a lifeway of constantly challenging myself to grow and expand beyond the limits of my vertiginous body.

Since the mid-seventies I have focused on helping others, as I have had to reinvent my goals based on the on-going reality of MS. Today as an author, college professor, and a volunteer for the NPS, I have realized that only by helping others to understand their personal value and worth through the power of education and faith in oneself can I repay the gift I was given at birth, the creative voice of a writer. At this time, 2001, I have 14 published books, of fiction, nonfiction and video documentaries as well as natural history books for the NPS.

This book crystalizes my philosophy concerning the challenge of living daily with my chronic disease companion by remaining positive concerning the roller coaster ride

I'm booked on for the remaining days of my life. My poem
says it best.

> *In the Dance of Health*
> *The eastern clouds sing*
> *With a message today:*
> *It is the enemy within*
> *That we must see through.*
> *It is the friend outside*
> *That we question and learn from.*
> *Together only are we whole.*
> *Together only can we dance*
> *To the music of history*
> *Weaving the fabric of reality*
> *Into harmony, offending only*
> *Emperors, Tyrants, and Disease. MVM 1994*

PREFACE

Dear Friends:

I decided to write this book because it seemed the only way I could share the growth I've experienced over the past 30 years in dealing with Multiple Sclerosis (MS) and its hidden disabling features. Through research, creative visualization, positive thinking, and strong faith in myself, plus the optimistic reinforcement of my support group, I have managed the first thirty years of my disability with courage, and a 'don't quit' attitude.

During the past years I have lived with daily reminders of this disease. Most of the time, I could ignore the symptoms, but not always, and not without multiple hospitalizations. Each step along the path of recuperation has brought me more solid evidence of the importance of never giving up, no matter the disability, and remaining open to alternative treatments. This is the element I want to share with you, the reader. Always think you can be the best you can be, despite obstacles, and the judgment of others. Believing in yourself is the key. For it is you and you alone who must master the living reality of the disability, and go on.

I have remained physically active, and though I often walk with the MS gait (dragging one foot), most of the time, no one can tell I am a victim of this young adult illness. Part of my success in not succumbing to the disease is by keeping my mind busy is due too constantly challenging myself to grow and expand mentally and emotionally beyond the limits of my body. I want to clarify here that each individual's progression with MS is different, from the symptoms, to the causes of the attacks. My progression is uniquely mine. But, because my symptoms are classic MS, I was forced early to accept the condition and do something constructively about it on my own. What I did has worked for me and I offer it to you in the hopes that some parts of it might work for you too. I have found positive methods that have kept me walking and enjoying each day, so far.

The times I am filled with discouragement and tears are the times I've found I must seek my *Inner Circle of Health*. I must look deep within myself and reaffirm my values, seek awareness of alternatives to the reality of my condition and the support of my conferences. This step has been tedious and often repetitive, but slowly I've found answers that I've decided to use on a daily if not hourly basis.

These answers are often outside the normal realm of western science and medicine and include prayer, acupuncture, nutrition, vitamins, Herbs, holistic medicine, positive visualization, and reduction of stress in my work-a-day world, as well as in my play-world. Also, I seek out the companionship of individuals who are themselves seekers of self-knowledge and inner strength.

It is hard to give up what feels most comfortable to one's self. Yet the results are so superior to the normal reality of Multiple Sclerosis progression that I've stepped within the embrace of the alternatives without even noticing when or why I left the folds of the routine. This is not to say that I've abandoned western medicine; I have not. But I've found that though traditional western practices have great diagnostic tools and often, amazing drugs to keep the disease in check, they often lack insight into possible alternatives that are reliable and effective, and less expensive in the overall repression of the symptoms of this disease.

I have always felt that anything that gives *us* an edge over a disability should be used gratefully and shared generously with those seekers willing to keep an open mind, and make it work for themselves. Most of this book was taken from my diary of recorded events that have changed my life. My view, and the techniques I learned through research and putting the challenge to the test are all steps along the path to trusting me. For me the method worked, and it has helped those who have copied the same techniques that I have worked with.

I have shared with professional therapists, support classes, and groups refining my techniques and skills through the years. As a college instructor I have attended or taught classes, sharing the skills with MS victims and friends. In the last few years I have found the Edgar Cayce Wet Cell appliance that combines spiritual healing with down to earth science. This unique appliance works with the electrical fields that surround the body, balancing the immune system within the electrical energy of an individual. This distinctive treatment helps to bring the electrical impulses into harmony allowing the synapses to be recharged and function again. I have watched the positive results of each visionary's insights—western, eastern, and spiritual—as others use these insights, and myself they bring us each the strength to deal with MS. I have also discovered skull acupuncture, Electromagnetic treatments including the Rife Tool and the Magnet Nikken products these have been critical to my maintaining my overall stability.

I do not consider myself an expert on the art of positive thinking. I am, rather, a student of the subject and the more I study and use this technique, the more I discover how vast is its potential. Positive thinking goes by several current doctrines and includes Creative Visualization, self-hypnosis, and self-love. It incorporates belief systems, religion, philosophy, and an individual's mind. Psychological awareness is an way to start self-help treatment.

My sources are many. I've included at the end a list of books, tapes and nutritional guidelines including a herbal pharmacopoeia that may aid the reader in understanding and studying this phenomenon and making the philosophy of self-health a part of each day's living experience. I've included sections on nutrition, spontaneous remission, modern drugs including the ABC drugs now used to keep MS in remission; i.e. Copolymer—1 Betaseron, Avonex, Copaxone, Interferon, and Nantune. As well as electromagnetic treatments including the Rife Electromagnetic Tool and the Magnet Nikken products discovered and used since the 1930's as well as vitamin therapies and Doctor Valerie Hunts meditations and exercises. This diary is my gift to you, my reader. I hope it helps to open one set of eyes to the reality that an incurable condition is only that if you let it be so.

Remember that the simple ingredients of good health are so logical that we often take them for granted. These ingredients are: good nutrition, adequate rest, and ample exercise. By consciously remaining positive in thoughts and actions, dreaming positively, and keeping your mind open to the possibilities beyond the physical restraints of a disease that can be disheartening, demoralizing, and debilitating, your life can remain fulfilling, happier, and more active than you ever dreamed possible.

In conclusion, I wish to acknowledge three of the individuals who have offered their support and encouragement through the years. My husband, Ken Mabery, deserves special recognition for his faith and support of me through the 30 years we have been together. I wish to thank Doctor of Oriental Medicine, Gerald Dukeminier, Doctor Jason Hao, my Acupuncturist's and for their selfless contributions to the finished text and their willingness to teach me the founding principles concerning the ancient art of acupuncture so that I can perform this ancient art on myself. Judith Andreica, M.Ed., LPC counselor and friend who has graciously offered insights into stress management and support in the first forward with Dr. Dukeminier.

The prelude perceptions are from my Acupuncturist and psychologist of ten years. Their combined insights within the Forwards are evidence of what may lie beyond our limited daily understanding of our body and its interconnected magnetic fields. I will state here that all that Mr. Cayce identifies is accurate to my life history. But at the time of occurrence, {the lightening events} between (1950's–1970's) either I was unaware of the specific results and power of magnetic fields or never put the two with the resulting condition of MS. On learning of the ground breaking research achieved by Doctor Valerie Hunt, with her award winning techniques in mind-field, energy research and consequentially finding self-healing techniques for breaking through Barrier diseases like MS she has introduced the phenomenal healing power of the scaler wave, and the need for consistency and faith in science on the cutting edge. Orthodox medical providers are questioning all of these techniques and tools at this time, but not dismissed and they offer possible amazing healing potential no matter the bodies present condition.

Today, I continue on a self-regime where I watch my diet, exercise, and emotional state. I have learned to recognize when I need help, what type of help I need, and I've learned to ask for it and receive it gratefully whenever it is given. This journey has been long and arduous with many surprises and pitfalls. I have learned to trust myself and make a conscious effort to maintain a positive attitude even on the days I feel horrible. This alone has helped to balance me so that I can deal with the bad days as well as the even worse hours that always sit in the shadow watching me as I have moved through them. I pray there is something within this text that speaks to you a fellow sufferer. I do know my research through the past 25 years has aided me in remaining positive about my future. I hope you too will find the strength to make a few of the suggestions work for you as well.

Joint Forward by Doctor of Oriental Medicine: Gerald Dukeminier, L.Ac And Counselor: Judith Andreica, M.D. L.P.C.

COUNSELOR'S FORWARD

An alternative title to Ms. Mabery's book might be, *If I Can Do It, You Can Too*. Her book is inspiring to all of us, whether or not we have a chronic disease. She has an indomitable spirit. She has taken pains to know herself. She strives to stay positive. She shares with others what she's learned, and become stronger through the process. All these are important to mental and emotional health.

Typical of her fighting spirit is her learning to do her own acupuncture. Her acupuncturist lived more than 140 miles away. Rather than give up and do without, as most of us might have, she asked him to teach her the basics of this ancient healing tradition. Also typical of Ms. Mabery is that she makes only passing reference to this in her book. Perhaps because her attitude of not giving up is so ingrained in her that she overlooks some of her achievements.

She also overlooked the inspiration that she gives to others maybe these others maybe long unaware of it too. The awareness sneaks up on them. After all, she is soft spoken and hardly talks about the challenges she must face every day. She seems much like you or me. So it can be surprising, after having known her for a while, to learn all that she has overcome. And continues to overcome daily, if not hourly. It is as through overcoming is now part of her psyche, and so she hardly notices it anymore. Just as the rest of us forget to notice the smaller stresses we face every day. Ms. Mabery has a longer view of time than most Americans do. "It stumped me for at least a year," she writes casually, when she talks about her struggle to become positive after her diagnosis of MS. A year seems little enough to begin to deal with any disease, much less a chronic one. Here one must think in terms of years, rather than weeks or months. It is a lesson for those of us who give up, if we don't meet our goals quickly or at all.

Another proactive stance she takes that would be healthy for all of us: She grieves what she has lost. Doesn't get stuck in the loss or the grieving but faces the passing of her former life, mourns it. Then she moves on to use crisis as opportunity. She resists the temptation for a stiff upper lip. She knows that too much stiffness can produce rigor mortise of the soul. She knows we need the softening of awareness and the acceptance of grieving before we can have the flexibility needed for the struggle.

What opportunity does crisis allow her that she might not have discovered otherwise? She gets to know herself. When we are pushed to our limits, we learn what's important, often making our old masks unnecessary, sometimes learning new ones. She learns the self-defeat of blaming and self-pity. She learns the challenge and joy of self-responsibility. She learns that in sharing her weaknesses with others, she watched, as they became stronger because of what she shared. In sharing we heal each other through exchange—with ideas that trigger our own faith. It bolsters our own emotional welfare and by giving we become supported. All these are lessons for all of us.

Ms. Mabery learned to walk "normally" by watching an ordinary woman. There is much to be learned from the ordinary. The convenience of our lives makes survival easy without having to notice things. She not only smells the roses. She recreates her life with them.

If we do only two things that Ms. Mabery recommends, our lives would be richer: Recognize the payoffs of our self-defeating behavior, and find our personal strengths. Often, the two are related. Even those of us who have achieved some of our dreams are still asleep when it comes to recognizing many of our strengths. Few of us have completely rid ourselves of negative thinking. And often, if we would go behind a negative thought, we would find a strength hiding. As Ms. Mabery says, it takes courage to use our strengths. Because, though negative thinking keeps us down, it keeps us safe. She has opted to give up the safety of being "sick," and invited her strengths in—teaching college, producing videos, writing books about her experiences etc.

Letting go of the "superficial appearance of health," as Ms. Mabery states, is good for all of us. Underneath our personae, who among us doesn't have some qualities that others might throw stones? I'm not suggesting we necessarily change what's underneath. But awareness of it, as she says, helps us become responsible. We are better able to use what we know for our advancement, and to preserve our relationships by not blaming our weaknesses on others.

If it's true, as Ms. Mabery states, that the reason for illness is that we learn to look and learn about ourselves, to test our awareness, is this not true of smaller trails? When we fail in our personal relationships or on the job, is our awareness not also tested? Multiple Sclerosis may be a test on a larger scale, but once again the lesson in becoming aware has meaning for us all.

Ms. Mabery's approach to her illness, which is really one of recovery and recreating, is a lesson for everyone. If she can remain positive and achieving with a disease of this magnitude, there is hope for the rest of us with our smaller challenges. As well as any of those with any other lifetime chronic disease her words speak to the heart. Perhaps that is the final lesson of this book—to rearrange our priorities. Perhaps what we thought was so divesting is not so daunting after all.

Judith Andrica, M.ED. LPC

ACUPUNCTURIST FORWARD Doctor Gerald Dukeminier, DOM, L.Lc.

From an esoteric point of view it can be said that all dis(ease) and suffering comes from not understanding that our identity is that of soul. We are spiritual beings having human experiences, seeking to rediscover our true essence. This spiritual journey to truth and beauty brings with it great suffering and pain. If we can raise our point of view to that of soul, we can then begin to value all of life's experiences as spiritual lessons and get on with our Divine evolution. Soul can instantly know the truth, but only when the casual, lower mental, astral, and physical bodies are brought into balance and harmony.

Health and well being can be defined as being in a state of balance and harmony within these love bodies. Marilyne Mabery in her book lovingly expresses her journey for winning the balance in her life. Her approach begins with the integration of body, mind and soul. She embraces an openness to create new possibilities for herself and others, and a willing acceptance of the process. Her search as led her to many new and exciting personal and medical discoveries.

One such discovery turns out to be several thousands of years old that of oriental medicine. Marilyne found it to be of great therapeutic value because of its integrated approach. The oriental model is based on the idea that no single part can be understood except in its relation to the whole, and views the whole as the complete physiological and spiritual, psychological faculties of the whole individual. She also discovered that she received the most benefit by keeping centered and focused on her inner self and by utilizing the best of both worlds of medicine, western and oriental.

In her book Marilyne illustrates that with an increased awareness of personal responsibility, of our true nature as spiritual beings bridges the gap between East and West, it brings benefit to the health and well being of mankind.

It takes inner love and guidance of our True Self and great personal commitment and sincerity to transcend the layers of mind, ego, emotions, and habitual patterns of behavior that separate us from our true essence. The faculties of thought, feeling, and personal will are powerful and important in healing but do not come close to the faculties of Soul which encompass freedom, love, power, wisdom, and Divine understanding. Even the most "incurable" "dis(ease) is "curable" if you seek its cause that lies within you.

Gerald Dukeminier, D.O.M.

ACKNOWLEDGEMENTS

To all of my friends and family who have struck by me through the highs and lows over the years. I must mention a few of these by name as they deserve special recognition, Ken Mabery, my husband who has given freely his phyical, financial, and emotional support for thirty years. Gerald Dukeminier, and Jishun Hao, Doctor's of Oriental Medicine for their treatments and concern through the early years of my journey and their unbending support whenever I arrived at their offices. Like all teachers these care givers generously offered their aid without knowing they made the difference for me by sharing their positive attitudes, knowledge, and belief in me as more than a survivor but a warrior on a life long quest in pursuit of health and a quality independant life. Nita Ford, my long time friend and consistant driver from 1995 until we transferred out of New Mexico in 2001. She alone knows the many tasks she performed unpaid except my unending gratitude. So many others were helpers along the way, they know who they are and how instumental in aiding my indepence and positive attitude. They each earned their Angel Wings each time they offered their help with strong hearts to keep me indepentant for thirty years.

LIST OF CONTRIBUTORS

Jerry Dukenminier, DOM, Jishun Hao, DOC, Judith Andrica,MW, LPC, Paula Bentley, LMT and Edgar Cayce.

LIVING WITH MS

CHAPTER ONE

The First Seven Months—Frustration
Fear—Anxiety
The Crisis—The Search for Facts

PART I

In 1974 my hands warped. This is the only description I can give to the oddity of my hands curling in upon themselves. My reality at the time of my first attack was that of a back-country park ranger in one of the most beautiful spots on earth. I was a college student with the goals of a medical career and a happy family life with my new husband. But suddenly my hands had curled into tight balls and it was minutes before I felt sensation back in them.

I couldn't understand why my hands would suddenly collapse inward at any hour of the day or night. I didn't understand why my speech suddenly slurred without reason. Nor did I understand why I was overreacting to things that normally would not have fazed me. Exhaustion haunted me hourly. I was only twenty-two. I had other problems during the previous two years. I had suffered from dizziness for a six-month stretch, from exhaustion, and memory loss. For these, still, I had firm diagnostic evidence of an inner ear infection, or at least the doctor thought so at the time. But now when my hands curled into tight fists and I tingled from head to toe, I began to wonder what I was doing to myself, or what was happening to me, and why.

I was happy with my life, my husband, my job, my studies, and the beautiful world that I was experiencing. But it was hot. Normal temperatures along the White Rim and Needles district of Canyonlands National Park in the early 1970's were one hundred plus degrees Fahrenheit in the summer, with nights cooling to the high eighties. With this extreme change in temperature in the summers and fall, rolling thunderstorms were an accepted reality. It was not uncommon for powerful lightening storms to knock out the park radio system, doing damage to other electrical items.

My work required that I be out in the sun eight to ten hours a day, hiking or driving jeeps over strenuous terrain. I had to deal with visitors in all types of situations; some stressful, some were life threatening health emergencies like rock rescues, or drowning, but most others were enjoyable. Prior to working as a park ranger, I had worked for six years as a student nurse in Carlsbad, New Mexico from age 13 to 18, while attending high school during the day and college at night or during summer sessions. This shows how highly motivated I was to succeed and how I ignored my age.

Because of my build, personality, and known family circumstances this young age factor was ignored by all the health professionals I associated with. I supported myself by nursing when I went elsewhere to college. I also married during this time, transferring and changing my major so that my husband and I could attend the same school.

At first I, we ignored the symptoms I experienced. Especially since the sensations were not perceived by others and usually lasted only a few minutes, or an hour, at most.

When I finally went to a doctor, he said I needed more sleep and less stress in my life. He prescribed Valium. I immediately had an allergic reaction or what I thought was an allergic reaction, and threw the drug away. My reaction to this relaxation medication was double vision. If you've ever experienced double vision you will understand that it is not only disconcerting but also immobilizing. Within a few days my vision returned to normal. I sought out more physicians and they were puzzled by my symptoms. One doctor thought it must be Meniere's disease, another thought it was a tumor on my spinal column, another nerves, or female problems leading to exhaustion. Three years had gone by since I had felt the first symptoms. In this time I had begun to doubt my sanity and definitely my health.

A move at this time occurred, from the Southwest I loved, to Theodore Roosevelt National Park in North Dakota. This was a place so dissimilar to my normal surroundings in New Mexico and Southeastern Utah that I might have been on the moon. We arrived in early October leaving behind the spectacular fall colors of Canyonlands National Park for a snowstorm. Within days of arrival a seven-day blizzard and twelve inches of wet snow inundated us.

Two weeks after this move I succumbed to a major attack of MS. We did not know it was MS then and I, of course, first thought it must be a stroke or a psychological reaction because I had not wanted to move.

For at least a week's time I was positive I was getting worse and I knew enough medicine to know that strokes are usually permanent, taking years to get over if one ever can. My self-diagnosis I soon learned was invalid, but my legs would no longer support me, my hands were useless, and my body tingled from head to toe now. I lacked energy even to read.

I attempted to disguise the condition from my husband. Because of the move and the new job it was easy to remain in bed and tell him I had the flu. Still, I knew better, after four or five days of remaining in bed until after he left for work, so he wouldn't see me crawling to the bathroom, he insisted on taking me to the doctor sixty miles away in the town of Dickenson.

Again, the doctor prescribed another sedative, this time Librium, though I had cautioned him about my first reaction to Valium. After I picked up the prescription I knew I would not take it. Actually, I was so angry with this man of medicine I flushed it down the commode. I knew my waffling limbs were not the result of nerves or even mental duress.

I put up a brave front, but again my husband carted me off to more doctors. These doctors were 750 miles away in Fargo, North Dakota. It was a teaching hospital with the State University affiliated with the Mayo clinic. The doctors did all their tests, including brain scans, x-rays, mylograms, and blood examinations, trying to sound positive for the five days I was there. But I had studied medicine in college and I knew the prognosis before they told me. Thankfully, the neurologist was willing to sit with me and explain what I could do to help myself with the disease's progression once he had identified the culprit as Multiple Sclerosis. Then he sat with my husband and me, explaining the realities of MS in clear professional English with compassion and heartfelt advice for the two of us.

We learned that MS, or Multiple Sclerosis is a disease of the central nervous system. It interferes with the brain's ability to control such functions as seeing, walking, and talking; also many others. It is called "multiple" because scar tissue or lesions effect many scattered areas of the brain and spinal cord. Symptoms can be mild or severe and come and go unpredictably. It is called 'sclerosis' because the disease involves "sclerosis," or hardened tissue, in damaged areas of the brain and spinal cord that interfere with the circuit/synapses that act as messenger carriers to the brain. Most healthy nerve fibers are insulated by myelin, a fatty substance that aids the flow of messages to and from the brain. With MS, the myelin breaks down and is replaced by sclera. This sclera distorts or even blocks the flow of messages to the brain. Often body functions become uncontrolled when the brain does not receive messages.

What causes MS is one of the biggest mysteries of modern medicine and science. Scientists have two theories. 1) *Virus Attack*: When virus attacks the body, it multiplies rapidly inside body cells. Most viruses cause symptoms quickly, others are slow growing and appear later. 2) *Immune Reaction.* Our bodies have a built-in defense system that destroys "invaders" like viruses and bacteria. This defense system can 'backfire' and start attacking the body's own cells; this is called an autoimmune reaction. MS might involve an autoimmune reaction where the body attacks its own tissues by mistake. Thus the high white blood cell count which MS individuals constantly have. 3) *Combination of both.* In this theory the body becomes confused because some viruses take over parts of cells—and the body might attack both host cells and viruses. The neurologist told us that MS is not a mental illness, nor is it contagious, or preventable or curable—yet!

Immediately the doctor suggested a change in diet for me: no more red meats, no more sodas, tea, or coffee with caffeine, eliminate caffeine completely, no more chocolate. Exercise was mandatory either with daily walks or in a pool where my body temperature would be regulated. This meant I had to learn to swim. I was never to get too hot; therefore, no aerobic exercising. Outside and inside temperatures were to be moderated. I was to manage my stress levels hourly; this meant for me, giving up my life-long desire to go into medicine or to work outside in temperatures above 90 degrees. I had to get and keep a positive attitude and make it live each day of my life.

And most importantly, I was to begin taking doses of Vitamin B, C, E, calcium and Lecithin, 19 grains four times a day all classic antioxidants. I was always to drink plenty of water, not tea or coffee because they are diuretics containing caffeine, and most importantly to avoid anything with caffeine.

The doctor spent some time identifying the many symptoms that I had not experienced yet, and he allowed me a glimpse of what might be in store for me if I did not take care of myself. He told me that symptoms vary greatly from person to person, even from time to time in the same person. These might include eye problems, double vision, or uncontrolled eye movement. Speech problems, such as slurring or stuttering could occur. Partial or complete paralysis of any part of the body was common. He forewarned of extreme weakness or unusual tired feelings, moodiness, and shaking of hands or limbs. Also, loss of coordination, loss of bladder or bowel control, numbness or prickling feelings in certain areas of the body or all over, and staggering or loss of balance, even obvious dragging of one foot, or the MS gait. A typical pattern is a short period of acute symptoms followed by an easing or disappearance of symptoms for weeks, months or even years.

** Note: Any of these symptoms could mean other illnesses—always check with your doctor.

As a would-be doctor, (my earliest aspiration was to be a physician and my early college studies were in medicine) I found his advice sound. The doctor led me to believe (or more appropriately, I believed) that if I made some of these basic changes I would be back to normal within a year. He emphasized that a diagnosis of MS is no cause for despair. MS patients do and can lead independent, active, satisfying lives in spite of occasional disability. MS, he told us, can be minimized with proper management. He suggested a coping mechanism, being counseling, to deal with any depression, anxieties, and limitations caused by MS and massage therapy.

Six months after adhering to the advice of the neurologist I was back to normal without taking any medication. At least what I thought was normal. I no longer limped like a drunken sailor. I was no longer tingling from head to toe. My hands had feeling again and I could hold a pen, without twitching at anytime. Nor was I crying at the drop of a hat. I lost weight on the new diet. My energy returned, and I felt better than ever before, positive this MS diagnosis had to be a mistake.

CHAPTER TWO

PART TWO: FARTHEST REACHES OF THE CONDITION
M.D.'s Point of View
Beginning Again at Twenty-five

The initial fear of this incurable disease for me was minimal. I had grown up in a home with a mother who was unhappy because she had excruciating back pain and other major health problems from the time I was a young child. She hardly ever complained. I didn't realize at the time this was a classic denial reaction on my part, based on my family history and would have to be dealt with at some time. Instead, because I had little pain, I could see no reason to fear the diagnosis when it came. Actually, I was elated to learn that the symptoms were those of a disease, rather than psychological in origin. During the previous two years, at least a dozen doctors had given me sedatives and acted confused by my complaints. This firm diagnosis was an opportunity and a blessing rolled into one. As I learned more about the disease I blocked all the unpleasant symptoms from my mind. And once I was back to normal, I quickly forgot the long-term effects of MS and, unfortunately, what was necessary to manage it.

Another move back to the Southwest occurred twelve months later. Our new job was in an extremely isolated area where phones didn't work with any consistency. Surrounded by the eerie beauty of Chaco Canyon in New Mexico, and without access to any type of support group, I basked for awhile in my naiveté. After my second full-blown attack two years after this move, and five days in another hospital with more tingling, vision problems, and weakness, I recognized my humanity, and the reality of living with MS. Still I did not put two and two together concerning the severity of this disease and the long-term stresses I had been under since childhood.

Once released from the hospital I went back to the daily regime of eating right, taking my vitamins, sleeping at least 8 hours a night, and cutting unwarranted stress from my life. This lasted six months, and again I was back too normal. This time, my emotions were still out of kilter, but not enough to be an embarrassment in public (for most of us, our worst self-inflicted fear is not looking good to others).

A year after the attack, I was back to my old routine of working long hours in a stressful office situation, eating poorly, forgetting about my vitamins, hardly exercising, and drinking caffeinated drinks. Most significantly, I became over-heated after a long hike and tried to cool off by drinking iced tea. At midnight, I, awoke with a sledgehammer between my eyes, and the most excruciating headache ever invented.

It was no surprise to have another five-day hospital stay. This time, and for the first time, I was given ACTH hormone and prednisone. Again I was given the advice not to get too hot, and to drink plenty of water, get enough exercise/rest, and do away with unneeded stress. I was to never become dehydrated again.

After reading all the information available at the time on steroids and their function in treating MS, I decided they were not worth the side effects at this time in my life even if they eliminated the tingling sensations and gave me strength.

This, of course, was a personal decision, but I would advise everyone to weigh the advantages and disadvantages of using certain medications to relieve the symptoms of MS. Ask your physician for his/her advice and then determine whether the benefits are worth the negatives that most drugs hold. The double-edged sword of drug use is an enigma each individual needs to be aware of. If the perceptions of those around you are such that you find *you cannot deal* with their judgments of you as a wobbling sailor, then, for a short time only, would I recommend the use of prescription drugs to alleviate symptoms. There are other ways to accomplish this, the rest of the text deals in detail with these.

After this hospital stay the advice stuck. Now I found I didn't have the information to understand or accept my condition. Nor did I have the insight to know how to help myself. I wavered for another six months before putting the first neurologist's advice to work. Again, I was soon back to speed, almost—only this time I was determined to be cautious and sought out every book I could find about the disease MS, also self-help manuals.

In the early 70's there were few books that I could find on this disease or even on nutrition. The few I found reaffirmed the neurologist's point of view, without giving enough detail to act as more than a guide. These included Adele Davis[1] books on

---

1. Davis, Adelle; *Let's Eat Right To Keep Fit* and *Let's Get Well* and *Let's Cook It Right*; New American Library, 1954

nutrition and eating right, John K. Wolf, M.D.'s work on *Mastering Multiple Sclerosis*[2]. And, I luckily discovered a hidden society, (hidden at least to me previously), the National Multiple Sclerosis Society[3]. Immediately, I sought out a counselor from the chapter in Albuquerque, and read everything they had to offer at the time. The only problem was that most, if not all, books of this period either dealt with the newly diagnosed, or the bedridden. Five years into the disease, I was still luckily outside both categories.

As I read these works, I realized that I was still on the outside looking in at the disease. My symptoms, though dramatic during attack periods, were not in physical evidence during my remissions, for the most part, I continued on with my normal life as if nothing were wrong. I remained mobile, active, and constantly seeking out more and more information to aid me with my condition. I tried to use what was currently needed and stored the rest until the day when I might require it. This, of course, meant that when the eventual event occurred, I forgot all I had learned until I could review my source material again.

A researcher by the name of Caryle Hirshberg wrote a report in the late 1980's concerning spontaneous remissions. In this landmark report he identified the 10 factors that indicate the individuals who, most likely will experience remissions in any disease[4]. These factors include: personal

2. Wolf, John K.; *Mastering Multiple Sclerosis: A Guide To Management*; Academy Books, 1975

3. Multiple Sclerosis Society, National Office; 205 East 42nd St. New York, NY 10017 (212) 986-3240

4. Hirshberg, Caryle: *Spontaneous Remission: The Spectrum of Self-Repair*, 4/1993; Noetic Science Review, Sausalito, California.

responsibility in caring for themselves; a feeling that they could influence the outcome of the disease; a feeling of purpose for their lives; unfinished goals; looking forward to the future; some type of physical fitness program; in general, survivors are assertive and can say "no", ability to nurture themselves by withdrawing from stressful involvements; they can talk openly about their needs and condition, active involvement with others with a similar condition.

During all my attacks I rarely battled depression. Instead of becoming depressed, I simply removed myself from the limelight and became more of a sideline observer than before, yet still involved. I know now that I suffered from the "not me" syndrome that is normal for any human facing a chronic ailment. This lack of acceptance was more understandable because it was rare that I displayed any outward symptoms that others, except those closest to me, would recognize.

Denial played a role here, not conscious denial, rather subconscious. If I didn't have to, I just didn't pay attention, nor did my husband. I did not grieve for the past healthy me because I didn't recognize the loss at that stage, nor did my husband. I did long for the stamina to get through my daily routine of living and I constantly sought out ways to cut corners so that I wouldn't wear out so fast.

My husband and I accepted this new me because it was a gradual change. I did know it was difficult for him not to have his companion when he wanted to get out and backpack the countryside or ski the slopes. Since I had never been very good at athletic endeavors it didn't concern me.

I did accept from the first diagnosed attack that I must be flexible with my career goals, and decided not to overburden myself with full time work or having children. It was only my superiors at work , who had a problem with my limited work availability, even after I sat them down and honestly detailed my physical limitations.

I began identifying the signs that forewarned of an impending attack, like exhaustion, moodiness, low energy, and concentration problems. I found that getting sufficient rest would often head off an attack. Still, my life was full of activity and often I just didn't pay attention to the signals.

I continued in my job for another nine months until I had another major attack. Once up and going again, I foolishly took another job in the same department that was just as stressful. The only difference was that I now worked for only one person, instead for a whole division. It took me awhile to recognize this as a pitfall in itself. Actually, it took me six jobs in six different fields of endeavor and eight more years of struggle with frustration and tears before I accepted the new limited me. During this time I regulated my work to part-time. I managed to remain ahead of the normal progression of the disease. Still I could feel a slow change in my self-confidence, also a new self-doubt surfacing.

I had been fortunate and never doubted or experienced self-doubts before the age of 22. In school I was highly motivated, I was a good student. I enjoy learning and sharing knowledge with others. In my jobs that included nursing, E.M.T., park ranger, administrative officer for a national park, CPA, and Financial Planning Assistant, I was normally the first to volunteer for a new assignment, new challenges. Now because of the exhaustion I had to stand back and watch others take over. It was a frustrating eye-opener.

Because of our National Park Service moves, another coin was thrown into my pool of adjustment. Everytime I established a support group of friends and co-workers, we moved, and I had to reestablish support all over. Only in the last years have I realized that I must accept the NPS (National Park Service) lifestyle as a challenge and look forward to the new area with enthusiasm and hope.

CHAPTER THREE

PART THREE

Getting Rid of the Anger
Healing Myself—Healing Meditations

Initially, I was not angry with anyone other than those doctors who had done nothing more than a quick physical exam and written me off as just another nervous woman. I was more frustrated and annoyed than angry that I could no longer participate in an active out-door life, or in medicine, my chosen occupation.

So what did I do? I worked to prove everyone wrong and when possible, went back to my old lifestyle, with only a whispering conscience to remind me of the facts.

It didn't take very long for the condition to rear its head with one or more of its many facets. Lack of coordination became a *role player* at this time, and I excused it because I had never been known as a graceful person. I laughed when I fell down and quickly learned how to fall 'softly'. Slowly, the intense heat of the Southwest began to affect me and I noticed that I had difficulty with emotional mood swings whenever I became overheated or tired.

What did I do about this? I began to blame my husband who refused to buy an automobile with air conditioning.

Because of our lifestyle and employment it seemed I could never draw the money together to purchase this luxury item to help myself[5]. I recognized an air conditioned car was a needed ingredient to aid me in keeping out of hospitals, especially since I had to drive 75 miles of dirt and paved road to the nearest town to buy groceries while we lived at Chaco. Life went on for at least 6 more years before I sacrificed and purchased the air conditioning unit for our car. And, before anyone, explained the IRS realities of tax deductions for necessary medical prescribed items I gritted my teeth and bore it.

During this time I had several minor attacks, from double vision to unbelievable mood swings. I also lost most of the sensation in the soles of my feet. I felt more body tingling, and many emotional upsets. These pushed away the most understanding members of my personal family: my husband, and even my pets. I was angry, but I didn't recognize my behavior or the results until I hurt my loving cat of nine years. Her stunned gaze, after I flung her across a room and her unforgiving manner from that day forward, stung me to the core. I then began to note the same expression in my husband, my parents, in-laws, and friend's eyes, also my job associates.

I went in for professional counseling for the first time and dealt more with my feelings of inadequacy in the job market than with my emotional turbulence with my loved ones. At this time I was instructed in the benefits of biofeedback. The following insights are from the book by Matthew J. Culligan and

---

5. IRS regulations allow any chronic disease sufferer to deduct the cost of equipment recommended by a physician.

Keith Sedlacek, M.D.: *How To Avoid Stress Before It Kills You.*[6] Biofeedback is a method that an individual can use to determine his stress quotient, also to learn methods for dealing with the stress in life. The "grandfather" of biofeedback is Neal Miller, who, in the 1950's and 60's, did work with managing conflict behavior, motivation, and social learning. Through this man's work, most formerly held beliefs about stress, changed. He showed that the autonomic system (the internal machinery of our bodies that controls visceral responses), previously thought to be beyond man's control, could be trained and reinforced with rewards to achieve balance within the framework of stress. This visceral learning was specific, that is, humans can change their heart rate without influencing other autonomic controlled variables, such as breathing rate, and blood pressure.

Miller stated in an article in *Science* magazine in 1969 that:

"Biofeedback should be well worth trying on any symptom, Functional or organic that is under neural control."

I have also included the 1990 stress scale in the back of this book. It is based on leading psychologist Georgia Witkin's, work *Social Readjustment Rating Scale for Stress in the 1990's.*[7] This, for me, identified more fully the new stress sources we as citizens of this great country did did experience on a daily, if not hourly basis.

---

6. Sedlacek, Keith, M.D. *How To Avoid Stress Before It Kills You*; Gramercy Publishing,
7. Witkins, Georgia; *Social Readjustment Rating Scale for Stress in the 1990's*; New York

Since MS is a neurological disease, this type of training is extremely helpful in dealing with cumulative stress. Starting a program of biofeedback training requires a knowledgeable physician or technician to take one through the basic steps while being monitored by the GSR, or Galvanic Skin Response, that detects stimuli that are important to the individual. This information is then fed through an electromyograph where both the individual and the technician can hear the audible decrease of the neurological reaction to stress. This feedback loop creates an ideal learning situation for the individual, helping us to recognize the impact of stress upon our bodies. By using EMG training, an individual can experience states of muscle relaxation far deeper than those experienced by others in their everyday lives.

What makes biofeedback training worth the extra commitment for an MS individual is that by mastering the methods taught in a relatively short period, I learned to alleviate the effects of cumulative stress on my body. The machines provided reliable, measurable information so that I was more aware of my body's function, and they showed the effect of my behavior on my body. By seeing that I could change what was happening, I was encouraged to play an active role in my well being. My only problem with this approach is that I must be alert to the signs and put this practice to work for myself as quickly as possible when a stressor becomes a factor in my daily routine.

Everyone feels stress. When handled properly, stress drives athletes and us to greater heights, greater achievements. Handled improperly, stress becomes distress. I learned that this can mean anything from exhaustion, nervousness, high blood pressure, chronic headaches, and other chronic disease complaints, to just plain misery. Before I tackled my next stressful session, I took a simple cumulative stress test given to me by my mental health professional in 1982.

Directions: Review the changes in your life over the past few months. Think about each question for about 30 seconds. Rate each. Remember: this is only a reduced version of the test.

1 = No Change 2=Little Change 3=Moderate Change

4=Considerable Change 5=Major Change

_____ Do you tire more easily?

_____ Do you feel fatigued rather than energetic?

_____ Are you working harder and harder and accomplishing less?

_____ Are you increasingly cynical and disenchanted?

_____ Are you often invaded by a sadness you cannot explain?

_____ Are you forgetting appointments, deadlines, personal items?

_____ Are you increasingly irritable? Short-tempered?

_____ Are you often disappointed in people around you?

_____ Are you seeing close friends and family less?

_____ Are you too busy to do even personal routine things?

_____ Are you suffering from physical complaints (aches, pains)?

_____ Do you feel disoriented when the activity of the day halts?

_____ Is joy elusive?

_____ Are you unable to laugh at a joke about yourself?

_____ Does sex seem like more trouble than it is worth?

_____ Do you have very little to say to people?

_____ Have you suffered an immediate family death recently?

_____ Have you had job difficulties in the past six months?

_____ TOTAL

SCORING:	0-25 You are doing fine
26-35	There are a few things you should watch
36-50	You are a candidate for cumulative stress
51-65	You are well into cumulative stress
65- +	You are a danger. You're physical and mental health are threatened.

After I received my initial rating in 1978 of 163%, the health worker identified for me a life event scale that signified each type of stress and its numeral ranking on a scale of 1-100. A sample of this scale follows. It will show you exactly where dealing with a chronic disease ranks amid all the other stresses of daily life[8].

RANK	SAMPLE LIST ONLY OF LIFE EVENT	MEAN VALUE
1	Death of spouse	100
2	Divorce	73
3	Marital separation	65
4	Jail term	63
5	Death of close family member	63
6	PERSONAL INJURY OR ILLNESS	53
7	Marriage	50

---

8. Witkin, Georgia; *Social Readjustment Rating Scale*; 1991

8	Fired at work	47
9	Marital reconciliation	45
10	Change in health of a family member	44

(Note this scale is a 1978 ranking. The updated 1998 List is included in Appendix A)

I now use this incredible tool whenever I am at my rope's end. I've learned its value. Still, it just hasn't hit home yet, that it is absolutely necessary for preservation of myself. This is shortsighted, I know, and yet we are each human, creatures of habit, and life is forever pushing us forward into new situations that take up our time, our energy, and our memory. I have purchased a small wallet card that I keep with me always. This card cost me all of a dollar ($1).

With this card I can quickly identify how much stress I am under. It is called a stress control card, or a biofeedback identifier. A bold strip is divided into four colors. Black is stressed, red is tense, green is calm, and blue is relaxed. All the card requires for a reading is that I place my thumb against a black pad for a count of ten. The color that appears reflects my current condition. On the back of the card an explanation is given concerning my results. When I am stressed, my blood is drawn inward causing cold hands, and the card will register black. If that happens, I try a quick relaxation technique until my card turns blue.

I recognize that if it's black or red now, I need to concentrate for some time to bring myself back into balance. I do this by resting, meditating, or doing something I enjoy. For a quick fix, though, I do the following to relax myself at once:

1. Clench my fists tightly for a count of ten. Release and let my body go completely limp.
2. Take a full deep breath and hold it for a count of ten. Exhale all at once, letting my body go loose and limp.
3. Breathing normally, let go more and more of my conscious thoughts, let out each breath as I count from 20 to 10.
4. Imagine myself basking in the warm sun on a beach, or soaking in a hot tub until I can actually feel the warmth in my hands.

LESS STRESS ACTIVITIES
SMILE AT OTHER PEOPLE.
LAUGH AT MYSELF.
THINK OR DO ONE THING AT A TIME.
RECALL PLEASANT MEMORIES FOR 15 MINUTES.
LISTEN TO MUSIC WITHOUT DOING ANYTHING ELSE FOR 15 MINUTES.
CHEERFULLY say "GOOD MORNING" to my family and to the people I meet.
CAREFULLY, SLOWLY scrutinize a tree, a flower, a sunset, or a dawn through a window or in my mind's eye.

FAMILY ACTIVITIES
SPORTS ACTIVITIES   CAMPING
HIKING   ACTION ORIENTED
                           MOVIES
AIR SHOWS   SHOOTING GAL-
                           LERIES
ARCHERY GALLERIES   MINIATURE
                           GOLF/GOLF

BOATING, SAILING, SWIMMING   READING
YARD OR GARDEN WORK   RODEOS
MOVIES   MUSIC CONCERTS
MUSEUMS, CITY—STATE—NATIONAL PARKS
PLAYING BOARD GAMES

EIGHT WAYS TO DEAL WITH STRESS

1. Strenuous physical exercise alternating with relaxation will alleviate some physical reactions to stress.
2. Structure my time. I keep busy. I do things that feel good to me. Reach out to others. Talk to people—they do care! Talk can be the most healing medicine.
3. Remind myself that I am normal and experiencing normal reactions to a stressful incident in my life. Don't label myself "crazy".
4. Keep my life as normal as possible. I don't make any big life changes.
5. Avoid alcohol and drug use. Don't complicate my feelings with a substance abuse problem.
6. Help my co-workers by sharing my feelings and seeing how they are doing.
7. Give myself permission to feel rotten, and don't try to hide my feelings.
8. I watch my diet: avoid sugar and caffeine. Eat regularly, don't skip meals.

I must mention that as humans we expect certain things in this life. One is health and another is love. The next is appreciation from others for our unique abilities, and respect for those exclusive talents. Even the most sensitive soul is less than awake when reality hits them flat in the face with a chronic illness. There is a Universal Law that states, "No one believes it can happen to him or her until they can't lift a finger to change their life situation."

This is yet another mistake in my history. I followed the path of error by justifying my apparent wellness by thinking I just didn't need to do anymore to remain healthy. Most times I felt good. I closed myself to the facts. When I felt bad, I felt worse because I knew inside, what was happening was because I was no longer in control of myself. Even so, the myth that because I had been diagnosed with MS, I wouldn't attract any other ailments was alive within me, though rationally I recognized this as plain foolishness.

This time though, rather than acknowledging that it was myself I should take to task, we moved. I blindfolded myself again blaming everything on the NPS lifestyle that is often unsettling and preoccupied with dynamic change in personnel. Like the military, Park personnel move on the average every one to three years, throughout their thirty-year careers. This means that the adult partner or significant other of the marriage team with the chronic illness (the one not a career participant in the NPS) also moves, and relocates, and must adjust to a new environment. This will include new neighbors, political realities, new locale, job parameters, and friends. This is unsettling even for normal, healthy individuals. Place a chronic disease in the illustration and you have a burning powder keg.

For years I did not realize this, and I know that even now my husband is only beginning to adjust to the actuality; the most important thing here is that we have both finally accepted the reality and taken steps to maintain ourselves in a healthy relationship without compromising our life-goals, or ourselves. Instead, we have each adjusted, sought alternatives, support groups, and activities together that build our individual self-esteem, and confidence. This keeps us, motivated and in love. It takes constant work and the ability to compromise but it can be done if the partners are firm in their commitment to each other and their basic principles are interwoven.

But at last, I recognized the anger within myself and the sorrow I felt at losing touch with the active world that I thrived in before MS became a factor in my life. Still I wouldn't admit, to anyone except myself, that this part of the reality was valid and needed attention. I didn't even have a name for what I had identified. I felt that I was to blame for making such a mess of my life. I felt isolated and of no importance to the world. I began to wonder why I couldn't get anything done even to my satisfaction, not to mention others'. The anxiety I felt was unspoken and unshared as I became more closed to the outside world.

Homeopathic medicine was introduced to me from several sources about this time in the 70's. Homeopathic medicine is a growing realization that often the best medicine is the medicine of taking care of oneself. I had learned what my body required for health. And a friend suggested herbal teas as a possible solution to my flexing emotions. I tried these and found soothing results from Chamomile, and Sleepy Time teas; as well as others. These teas can now be found in most supermarkets today, but then, in the early 70's, I had to locate a health food store. Another friend asked if I had ever tried meditation. Since I practiced yoga, I easily took up fifteen minutes of meditation a day.

Another friend, suggested alternative medicines including herbs and massage therapy, and most recently, in 1993, the Cayce Wet Cell that was envisioned by Edgar Cayce a century ago. This ingenuous mixture of chemicals and electromagnetic fields is so simple and yet so powerful I feel anyone with any type of neurological problem will benefit by investigating and trying this inexpensive method of treatment[9]. The process is a battery type apparatus that you or I connect yourself to after mixing the proper chemicals into a solution box. Then for the next half-hour just relax and allow your mind to drift or meditate. In using this simple technique in 1994 I encountered the following message that appears in the accompanying text as the Edgar Cayce channeled message. Whether the information channeled is from deep within my psyche, or was channeled through the great master, all I know is that it has brought me a new balance and awareness of the importance of all I share in this volume.

The following information in the treatment section was channeled to me in April 1994 while I was in trance. It is from Mr. Edgar Cayce (the sleeping prophet who died in the 1940's) while I was attached to his Wet Cell Appliance. Mr. Cayce was a devout Christian and developed the astounding ability to enter a self-induced trance in which he could diagnose illnesses and

---

9. Cayce, Edgar; *Wet Cell*; A.R.E. Clinic, Pathways to Health, Phoenix, Az. 1-(602)-955-9206.

prescribe treatments for individuals he had never seen before, sometimes thousands of miles away. When he died in 1945 he left behind a legacy of over 14,000 "readings" all of which are on file at the Association of Research and Enlightment, 67th Street and Atlantic Avenue, Virginia Beach, VA 23451; A.R.E. Press 1-800-862-2923. He envisioned the Wet Cell appliance for treating MS while he was alive in the early part of the 1900's. His words are accurate concerning my present condition and his insights have aided me in understanding some needed therapies I must pursue and the frequencies and vibrations of disease and the art of treating a chronic problem with consistency and faith.

EDGAR CAYCE—THE SLEEPING PROPHET CHANNELED MESSAGE TO MARILYNE MABERY 4/94

During the dark hours of the soul, while it was searching for peace I found this young woman who was requesting aid from the spiritual realm and began to channel information to her concerning the reality of her condition and what she could do for herself and others to regain her bodily balance. The medical profession has titled the symptoms she displays as those of Multiple Sclerosis. Having experienced this condition while I was alive, in others, including their lack of coordination due to loss of balance and strength, I've watched many endure this condition with no hope of ever regaining their former vitality. It is a sin for the young to be thrown this debilitating condition that should be reserved for the extremely old or no one at all. Yet, the lesson this disease teaches is one of the most powerful and meaningful ever written. Though the western medical reality has to do with medicines that are chemically made, my answer has to do with something even more powerful and long lasting. The body is made up of chemicals, yes, and chemicals can aid it in regaining and maintaining harmony in some cases. But the body with MS is out of balance for an entirely different reason.

The human body also is made of neurotransmitters and synapses. The body is electric and must be treated as an electrical energy field. Once the electrical field is damaged, either through disease or massive electrical or magnetic disturbances then the symptoms displayed maybe those of MS or any other neurological disease that baffles a traditional organic doctor. Anytime the neurological body is involved look to an electrical dysfunction caused at some distant point in the patient's life, in some distant part of the body. As each body has different tolerances for foods, so each body responds differently to electrical or magnetic energy. Of course the symptoms may be complicated by other less distinct items including, culture, age, stress levels, psychological realities, and nutrition.

In the case of Marilyne, she has been within structures that have been belted with lightening on several different occasions. Once as a child (recall the shock at the kitchen sink), once in a ranger station (recall the sizzled radios and your prone position afterward as the thunder rolled by), and several times within your home when lightening storms revolved over them. Each time the result to the electrical mechanical items within the structures was destruction. To the human body a combination of things happened, including sizzled nerve endings, and blown synapses within the spinal cord that extended outward into the organs and brain. Often the subject's reaction was not instantly obvious, other times in her case, it was ignored. Sickness resulted that was explained through guess work, either by herself, or a less than experienced practioner who did not connect the electric power of the storm to the magnetic reality of the human organism.

Now her condition is complicated through chemicals that are used with the best of intentions. These chemicals include Solumedrol, Aspirin, and vitamins, Steroids—including ACTH and Prednisone. These relieved the obvious bodily symptoms for a short times, (recall the difference in time to spirit and human reality) but the underlying cause has never been addressed.

By aiding the body with good nutrition, stress relieving exercise, and acupuncture the individual has been able to maintain her in a superior fashion for twenty years. But as all bodies do, they age, and one with a chronic disease, ages swiftly, even with the best of care. One's attitude aids the individual since they see results eventually. She has experienced improvement at every juncture of her journey. She has recognized and commended herself for doing the best she could do with the resources available.

She has never resisted her treatments, and, if anything, accepted them as part of her normal everyday life. But she has often overlooked heat and cold temperatures as an agitator of her neurological net. She is the daughter of a diabetic and hasn't monitored her blood sugar, though she has been aware of it since childhood. The life choices she has chosen are normal within the free-will zone of her life. Awareness of the food chemicals within her diet will awaken her further to the importance of monitoring her day-to-day activity. By cutting the excess sugar, caffeine, and chocolate she will feel stronger with fewer symptoms.

As for the monthly period of hormonal fluctuations, the culprit is too much estrogen. The body cannot compensate for the sudden excess and therefore the corporeal weakness. This will improve only with awareness of medical care-givers that can address it, check the dates before and after the weakness. Look for signs of restlessness, mood swings, and lack of balance while walking to identify this event. They will remain of short duration. Take precautions during this period. This is a time when physical injury may occur.

The positive results Ms. Mabery has experienced by using my Wet Cell Appliance, my channeled vision, are a combination of adjusting her electrical energy fields, combined with using the Crystals' therapy she has discovered. With Acupuncture she has found part of the solution for herself. The skull acupuncture is able to reconnect the synapses in her brain and allow for short-term agility. Unfortunately this method is limited by the treatment method. But by maintaining a treatment schedule she now knows when she is pushing the limits of her body and when she needs outside aid in transforming the reality of weakness to strength. She also recognizes, through helping others understand the condition and taking positive steps of action, that they may relieve themselves of many damaging realities of this disease. She also believes with all her heart and soul that she can and has experienced a cure. All she needs today is energy and belief in herself to rebuild her body to its youthful stamina. By identifying and maintaining the magnetic fields of her body, the Chakras will remain awake and stay within their balancing meridians. By incorporating new knowledge like the psychic healing technique of the Scaler Wave* discovered by Dr. Valerie Hunt she will burst out of the stall she has been trapped in during the past stressful years since 1998.

Only through accepting the lesson for what it is, a learning process, has she maintained herself and grown. Her electric body still needs work, since awareness of this was only begun on 4/94. Other answers will come to her, so that she may help others also. As she meditates and attunes her cells to the new energy level that is now aligned she will experience positive tensile strength in her muscles and organs. The stage is set, and the audience is primed.

The electrical magnetic body is what I'm addressing here. The human body is a master-computer with circuits that resonate power and energy. Every part is interconnected and needful of every other part. For the MS sufferer the parts have become isolated too long, in essence, they have atrophied. To regain their function they need a jump-start, either by another bolt of electric juice through physical awareness, or one of therapy.

Since magnetic therapy is not readily available at this time for her, or to others, she will have dreams that will allow the development of the appropriate devices. Many of the devices are being "envisioned as I write this" by others, but they will not know what to do with them. Resistance by Marilyne to this fact will be humorous, since the knowledge will come in dreams— via her subconscious—answers will arrive with precision and specific information. Without this complete information the devices she and others will create will be useless. Those who understand will appear, not as coincidence, but as scheduled, as I have. EC {Channeled Message to Marilyne V. Mabery 4/94 From Edgar Cayce}

NOTE TO THE READER:

Cayce once noted to a user of the Wet Cell: When the appliance is used, let that be the period of the mediation. Lie prone, or almost so, when it is used; and not let the mind run hither and yon, but let the mind be rather in the constructive way and manner. For as the mind and body and the soul are the triune, so there is the feeding of the spiritual self in the ways and manners as the physical body is fed—by thought. For the mind is the builder, and as the soul thinketh so it is.

Then during the period let it be in that attitude of constructive hopefulness, and know—no medicine, no application, and no mechanical appliance or otherwise, does the healing—but that only by the attunement to the divine within brings health. [261-27] [10]

Contact the Cayce Foundation in Virginia Beach, Virginia 1-800-273-1112 for further information concerning this man's insights and treatments.

An idea that grew out of all the others was that preventive medicine is really only an emphasis on the creation of health by each individual. The creation of health within the individual, who is out of balance in some way, requires more knowledge and understanding than I had available in the mid '70's.

In the early '80's stress was not a subject of daily conversation, nor was nutrition, at least not in the group I was associated with. Health food stores became my source for books

---

10. Cayce, Edgar; Wet Cell Appliance; [528-6] & [261-27]

and other material on nutrition. By changing my diet dramatically I immediately saw positive results that gave me a sense of false confidence.

Again, I justified my apparent wellness by thinking that because all these things had worked I really didn't need to know any more about myself. What a fool I was and still am to a degree. At last I have recognized that healing myself is a minute-to-minute job, and I cannot take advantage of myself or make excuses for my behavior. No one pays for it more than I do. I have recently been introduced to the groundbreaking work of Doctor Valerie Hunt. Her intriguing work is with the bio-electronic fields the human body creates in wellness and in sickness. Her identification techniques rely on intense measurements that are subjected to scientific scrutiny. Her books, *The Infinite Mind* and the companion workbook, *Mind Mastery Meditations* take normal mediation to the next step, integrating the mind and spirit upon a wellness quest unparalleled in the literature. I highly recommend anyone seeking insights into the higher level of meditation to seek out her techniques and make them a part of any wellness plan. They work and have made a monmental difference in my over all health and awareness in 2000.

Unfortunately, it was eight years after my initial attack before anyone even suggested the ancient art of acupuncture. This process looked interesting to me, and since I had no phobia concerning needles I decided it would be worth a try, except at the time, finding an acupuncturist was almost impossible.

Not until we moved to Santa Fe, New Mexico in 1987, fourteen years into my disease, could I find a therapist who practiced this ancient art. My first appointment was with an acupuncturist named Makima. She quickly relaxed me and after a lengthy interview took my pulses, first on my left side, then my right, and then at my throat. She explained this mysterious process as akin to tracking an elusive cougar. She asked if I understood how Aspirin worked, and when I shook my head no, she continued, "Is it of interest how Acupuncture works since it does work?" I supposed not, and yet my curious nature led me to begin reading all I could find[11, 12, 13].

The pulses are the most important tool of diagnosis for correct treatment of an individual with acupuncture. Unlike western medicine, she did not require blood samples or lengthy lab reports or days of hospitalization. Instead, she began treatment right away. She started by inserting thin painless needles in my legs and feet, and applying moxa herb to the needles on my right hand and my legs. During this half-hour she put on some relaxing flute music and encouraged me to relax and if possible, go to sleep.

Within one appointment I regained partial feeling in the soles of my feet where all sensation had been missing for over two years. My emotions became controllable after my third appointment, and tears became an infrequent normal release of the stresses of my life. The results of these initial appointments were immediate and so dramatic that I now have a standing appointment with my Japanese trained acupuncturist in Albuquerque. About every six weeks I go

11. Connelly, Diane M. Ph.D.; *Traditional Acupuncture: The Law of the Five Elements*; Center for Traditional Acupuncture, Inc. 1980

12. Cerney, J.V.; *Acupuncture Without Needles*; Parker Publishing Co., 1988

13. Griggs, Rick; *Personal Wellness*; Crisp Publications, 1989

in for a tune-up, unless I'm undergoing intense stress or common illnesses.

I will forewarn all readers that acupuncture generally requires multiple appointments before any lasting effects are induced. My immediate success lasted only briefly, but now with a regular schedule of treatments I find I can maintain myself well.

Traditional acupuncture, either Chinese or Japanese is based upon understanding nature as expressed in the human animal. Acupuncture originated in China about 5,000 years ago. It is a complex system of examination, diagnosis, and treatment. The healing art of Traditional Acupuncture, I found, requires years of study, and is rarely addressed in the cookbook type articles one reads in the western magazines and through our media. The grounding principles are reflected in the Law of the Five Elements[14] as viewed by the Chinese philosophy. These elements are: WOOD, FIRE, EARTH, METAL, and WATER. I am classified as WOOD, this means that certain points are effective in treatment for me with my condition. These include: points on the kidney, liver, and spleen meridians as well as others. The kidney points are most effective in producing immediate remission of symptoms in me. Other individuals, of course, will find their disease progression involves any of the other four elements, and this will be up to the individual acupuncturist to decide.

After the therapist believes he/she has adequate information concerning the patient's condition, the treatment can

---

14. Connelly, Diane M. Ph.D.; *Traditional Acupuncture: The Law of the Five Elements*; Center for Traditional Acupuncture, Inc. 1986

begin. First the pulses are taken. I use the plural because the practitioner must take the twelve pulses to determine the root of the problem, and if the oral interview information is accurate, and if any information is left out. Within these few minutes the therapist is also noting the color of the patient's skin, the fingernails, and tongue.

Once this is completed, needles are inserted according to the needs of the patient. Treatment varies, but it is a good rule of thumb that after the initial treatment patients respond optimally by being treated twice weekly, until most of the pulses maintain their balance. Dramatic change will occur within the patient. This leads to an awakening sense of well being and slow realization that this is probably the best they've felt in years, perhaps in their whole life. A system of follow-up therapy can be set up once the patient is stable. Patients are asked to come in for seasonal "tune-ups" for preventive measures. During these follow up appointments the long-term needs of the patient can be achieved. With chronic illnesses and the depth of the condition it may take longer for an individual to reach the optimum level of health. By following daily dietary and lifestyle recommendations this will bring one back into a state of balance. With *courage*, and a positive attitude the *rate* of recuperation will be shortened and maintained.

Still, I had psychological symptoms I could not explain, or understand, and did not realize that the ancient art of Acupuncture could help me by balancing these out as well. Finally, one afternoon, I went to the silence of a beautiful canyon and sat on a sheer cliff and screamed until I no longer had a voice. I screamed at fate, at stress, and at the unfairness of this rotten disease. Afterward, I sat there and cried at the loss of the possibilities that had motivated my life and felt sorry for myself. Then a tailless lizard slithered past and lifted itself on its one remaining leg to bask in the glory of the afternoon's warmth. Suddenly, I saw myself in that little creature.

Normalcy crept in again. I realized that I'm not alone in my struggle to maintain my life. I had known this since childhood in watching my mother, and later working in hospitals. Still because it was *me*, I had avoided accepting all the excellent advice I had sought out from the medical profession, feeling that they had let me down repeatedly. I went back to a counselor, after years of leading a pretty normal life, and asked pointedly why I had the feelings of inadequacy I have described to you.

The first issue we dealt with was the grief I had never allowed myself to feel because of losing my health. Finally I accepted grief as a universal experience. Each person's grief is individual and depends on their upbringing and previous experience. Because I grew up in a dysfunctional family (my mom was ill and became a prescription drug addict when I was seven), (my father was an off again/on again alcoholic by the time I was ten) I became what is termed a classic co-dependent that never placed myself first. I have always been an over-achiever, striving to help others by making them proud of me, but never seeming to succeed. Grief and anger were things I had avoided. Now I learned that all individuals have similar reactions to grief, even when they do not realize they are grieving. Most of us experience grief in varying degrees when faced with a loss, such as a loved one, or the loss of an illusion we've cloaked ourselves in so that we can deal with reality as we perceive it. This refusal to acknowledge grief I learned is only another type of denial.

I learned there is a pattern to human grief that is inevitable. There is anger, hurt, pain, fear, depression, and a feeling of loss. Grief is not a weakness, nor a lack of faith, but is a physical and psychological necessity. We cannot not grieve.

Grief, for whatever reason, with its many vicissitudes lasts far longer than our society recognizes. It is a natural yet complex process that includes love, anger, frustration, fear, bewilderment, and loneliness. Grief is cathartic and therapeutic. As I talked over my experience, the pain decreased and with it, the self-blame. In fact, most of my grief reactions diminished in severity by themselves. I found I had resources within myself that enabled me to recover from traumatic experiences not only in my past, (for example my lost childhood), but now even that of my health. I found that by identifying my losses I allowed myself to gain important insights. By facing myself I recognized my priorities and placed a perspective on my goals and achievements. It allowed me to experience my real and deep feelings more intensely. This seeing and experiencing was important in my total recovery and growth.

To live through grief I had to allow myself to cry freely or to exercise until I felt a release of tension. I found I should only drink juices or water and eat small meals while I was upset or until my gastric distress diminished.

I found rest essential, even if I could not sleep. When I couldn't sleep I read or did something I considered physically relaxing. I knew to use medication sparingly and only with the advice of my physician. I avoided use of drugs and alcohol knowing these would only prolong or stop the grieving process. I put off major decisions such as quitting or changing jobs because of the high level of stress I was under. Whenever possible, I talked with friends or family members about my feelings of guilt. When no one was available I expressed these feelings on paper so that I could sort out what was real and what was self-blame. Here I learned to forgive myself for contracting the disease MS, and for handling my childhood the way I had.

I found that anger also can be shared with others by expressing it in healthy and acceptable ways, as through exercise, screaming in a private place, smashing old dishes or bricks, splitting wood, or pounding on pillows or nails, washing windows, wax stripping the floor, or repressing it with other distractions such as reading or watching TV. Most of these methods of expressing anger are physical and draining, but afterward I felt better. By seeking out alternatives, I found individuals who could help me preserve my identity and values that gave meaning to my life. In the midst of this self-work, I allowed myself to be grateful for my life, my family, friends and for the past life I mourned.

Now, thankfully, I have at last accepted the MS condition and am no longer angry with myself for failing to remain healthy like the superficial appearance of everyone else. Actually, because of this disease I have recognized how special I am. After 20 years with the condition I have proven repeatedly how different I am from the normal population, whether physically compromised or just plain healthy.

What makes me different? The best answer I can come up with is that I've been willing to accept and seek alternatives and I have accepted sound advice when it was given.

Alternatives include things such as acupuncture, vitamins, biofeedback, positive visualization, the Wet Cell as envisioned by Edgar Cayce a century ago, the Rife electromagnetic tool, the Nikken magnets worn on the body daily, support groups, counseling therapy, meditation, and a recognition that I have the ability and knowledge to continue to help others in their adjustment to this condition. Actually, I haven't lost anything instead I've gained much more than I would have had without this disease as my backer. My sensitivity was raised to a heightened awareness of others because of this illness. The empathy I feel for them is a part of me. I understand what other individuals are going through, why they may be rejecting their life when what they should do is embrace it.

The disease syndroms of fatigue and exhaustion are heady excuses that are unfortunately a real part of this disease. By recognizing that we have some control over our emotions is a big first step. We need to take ownership of our feelings and condition and not place blame on MS, our families, our employers, whoever. When we have low energy, fatigue becomes a factor in our reality. We become irritable and have less energy to make decisions and solve problems or to concentrate on anything for a period of time. We can become stuck in the cycle of emotions to the point where it is hard to get along with anyone much less ourselves. We are cheated out of full participation in life! First we need to recognize that we do have some control. I found the following suggestions work for me. You may too if you decide to take control of your situation.

*DON'T stay in bed. The more active you are the more you can do.

*DO Stay involved with friends, family events, recreation, life itself.

*If you can't do the activities you used to do, find some new ones.

*Learn the difference between *"earned fatigue"* (from an activity i.e. Shopping, walking) and fatigue from immobility (from doing nothing) and *MS fatigue.*

*Maintain a positive attitude. Try to think about other things besides MS. MS won't go away by not thinking about it, but it won't be all consuming either.

*Develop some good support networks for yourself. Include groups, peer counselor programs, phone partners, and many other programs through your local MS Society.

*Communicate. No one can help you if they don't know what you need. Ask for what you need in a clear, direct way.

*Try psychotherapy: counseling can help and help you learn how to take control of your emotions.

*Learn relaxation techniques.

*Talk to someone when you are faced with a crisis or problem. Don't become a needy sponge, (a sure way to push family and friends away) instead offer your assistance where you can for their advice and help.

*Support others and your self*Have realistic expectations. Don't expect more from others because you are sick and disabled. *Try to give as well as receive.

*Learn to receive gracefully.[15]

---

15. Tinker, Mary. MS Chatter, 1995.

An introduction to meditation becomes a truly valuable one if you, the reader, have never practiced this ancient art. Meditation by definition is dwelling on anything in thought while awake and is most valuable in a relaxed state. It can also mean emptying the mind of all thought. There are innumerable types of mediation from prayer, to yoga, to deep breathing and visualization, to transcendental meditation. Each is valuable and easy to learn. I will recite only one type that seems to work best for me. This is the simplest I've experienced. It requires only that I be willing to make it a part of my day to day experience, and can be achieved in minutes in a hectic lifestyle.

Find a place that will be free of interruptions for at least fifteen minutes. Get comfortable in a chair or, if you prefer, on a couch or the floor. Loosen any clothing that may be too tight. Make yourself very, very comfortable.

Think of your bones and muscles and feel the weight of them on the floor on the floor or coach. With your eyes closed take a slow, deep breath. Exhale. Take a second deep breath, feel your body becoming heavier, the tension draining away. Exhale. Take a third deep breath, hold, tell yourself to relax. Exhale. Now as you breath deeply again, tense up your toes, your legs, your stomach, your chest, your arms and hands, your neck, your face, every muscle in your body. Hold for a count of five. Exhale. Feel all the tension you created in your body relaxing, unwinding, letting go. Feel all the tightness and tension of your day dissolving. Now, relax all your muscles a little bit more. Enjoy the release from tension. Feel the pleasant relaxing feeling spreading over your entire body. Hold that comfortable, pleasant feeling as you scan your inert body with your mind's eye. If there is a muscle that is not relaxed, tense it, hold it, then relax it. Your body should now be completely relaxed.

Let the pleasant sensation of relaxation flow through you from head to toe and back. Really enjoy this feeling. While you're relaxed you can give yourself some positive affirmations to carry with you throughout your busy day.

I can do this.

I am achieving my goals.

I pay proper attention to my nutritional needs.

My body is strong and healthy each minute of the day.

My mind works efficiently, effectively, and clearly.

I am supremely calm.

Each time you practice relaxing, it will become easier and faster for you. You will find that you can quickly shift into a relaxed state in which every muscle's tension drifts away. The more you practice, the more easily you relax. A few minutes of relaxation helps to relieve tension, fatigue, headaches and helps the mind stay alert, active, and better able to concentrate. To avoid monotony, mind-calming exercises should be varied from day to day. Besides additional mind-calming techniques already alluded to, mind-calming also can be done with cassettes such as *The Environment* series or relaxation records like *Spectrum Suite* or others you may find. Try a gizmo of the 1990's if the simple ones don't work for you, but whatever you do, make a daily resolution to yourself to spend five to twenty minutes a day relaxing.

Basic things one can do this minute are simple. Close your eyes and breathe deeply. Take six of these stabilizing breaths. Slowly exhale.

Now, still with your eyes closed, count slowly from ten backward, then open your eyes. I hope you felt some tension leave you.

Now stretch your back, lift your shoulders, hold your breath as you move. Exhale. Now you are ready to go back to whatever you were doing before, but now, a bit more in focus for your work whatever it may be.

Further things involve isometric exercises, including yoga relaxation techniques, biofeedback, and meditation at least twice a day when you first awake, and before drifting to sleep or whenever you feel yourself losing control[16].

You, as an individual, deserve to take sometime for yourself each day. As a person with MS, it is more important than you can believe. It is necessary. It is not selfish, not at all. Instead, by doing this for yourself, you become a more stable person who can advance through life touching others in a positive, uplifting manner. You will find more energy within yourself after you've made relaxation a steady habit.

Learn some basic coping mechanisms to encourage and support your new balanced lifestyle.

I learned a very important thing, once I identified my history and stress, to understand these different aspects, I had to tell my story so that true healing could take place. This meant that I had to shrug off convention and tell the truth of my life.

---

16. Hittleman, *Richard; Richard Hittleman's Yoga, 28 Days Exercise Plan*; Bantam Books, 1973

The miserable sections of my life, also the fun parts. Now that I have shared this with you, and my support group, I feel free to explore all the challenges my body decides to present to me. It is fun to realize that this disease no longer threatens me. Instead I'm aware of it and have learned methods to help keep myself stable and as close to remission as possible. I hope you too will find yourself beginning to recognize some areas you need to pay attention to and begin the emotional, psychological healing that is necessary to feel good about yourself and value yourself again.

Much of the work I needed to do was repetitive. I have recognized I will repeat myself often during this text concerning the varying skills I've had to learn and adapt to my daily regimen because through repetition only can anyone expect to make permanent change. Leading research has proven, *it takes an adult 21 repeated efforts* to make a lasting change in his/her life, see *How To Avoid Stress Before It Kills You*[17].

17. Culligan, Matthew J. and Keith Sedlack, M.D.; *How To Avoid Stress Before It Kills You*; Gramercy Publishing Co.; 1980

CHAPTER FOUR

Risk and Rewards—Plain Speaking
Where to Look—Outside—Inside
The Mission—Results—Good Nutrition—
Herbs—Yoga
Self-Esteem Is All Within

Think about what you are doing presently, its risks and rewards. What is your personal life like? Is it quiet or hectic? What is your family life like? Children scurrying around needing your constant attention, time stressed to the maximum, feeling guilty and exhausted? What are you eating, drinking? When are you eating? Are you able to get out and exercise? Or do you vegetate, hoping no one will see you stumble to the bathroom—can you +make it to the bathroom? Is it hot or cold where you live? Do you have any control over where you live? What is your self-image? What type of occupation are you trying to pursue? How many hours a week do you have to be professional? Do your friends, your spouse like you, or do you see yourself as the object of their pity? What are you doing to contribute to a healthy lifestyle in your daily, hourly life?

Think about what you would like to change. What is working, what is preventing you from moving forward? By evaluating your present condition and lifestyle against your desired goals you will lay the groundwork for perfecting a strategy for total wellness for yourself. Remember, you're of no use to anyone if you see yourself as not being useful even to yourself. Ask yourself these 7 questions. Write out your answers so that you can review them periodically because they will change, as all things do from time to time.

1. What are my dreams? What do I want to achieve in my life?

2. If I had one hour left to live, what memories would I have?

3. How do I spend my time?

4. What do I care passionately about?

5. From what areas in my life do I receive the most consistent positive feedback?

6. Do I view mistakes as learning opportunities or failures?

7. Do I have a good set of written goals to refer to frequently? If not, write them down—now.

I am not pointing a finger at anyone's present fitness being good or bad. Instead, I hope I am providing an avenue of information for you to evaluate, throw out, or use as you please. My goal is to leave you with a few insights and basics for developing your wellness idea and continuing to pursue the life long journey you are capable of traveling.

1. Eat a balanced nutritious diet. No more diet crazes with the pendulum effect.

2. Proper exercise must consider your present condition. Even deep breathing exercises are stress relieving. Try to walk or swim, exercise your limbs, it is all beneficial. In

water most MS people feel a freedom that is not available on land. Most can propel themselves gracefully for a few feet at least. It raises self-esteem and accomplishment levels to an all-time high.

I personally swim the length of an Olympic pool at least twice to six times. Then I back float two laps, then holding onto the side of the pool I lift my legs—one at a time for a count of fifty…to one hundred (I had to work up to this one). Then still holding onto the side of the pool I kick to a count of 100, or more if I'm not too tired. Then I swim two more laps if possible. I never exercise to the point of exhaustion, only until I feel tired. If I can't swim I walk a half-mile at least, farther if there is time and weather conditions are favorable. I did this daily in the summer months and at least once a month until 1999. We moved from NM that year and my daily exercise program took a backseat to balancing the move adjustment to maintaining our relationship to accepting more physical help from others, care givers, friends and family. Today in the December 2001 we have relocated again and I'm dependent on my physcal therapist, for the streaching he does with me and the pool work out I perform under his watchful eye. I'm dealing more and more with leg spasms, incontinence, and leg jerks. My new neurologist has upped the dosage on Oxbutynin, Baclofen, and I now take an antuipessantr, Celexa.

3. Seek out an impersonal support group. This can either be a therapist, an MS chapter support group, or a neighbor.

NOTE: a family member usually is too close to aid the individual with the chronic disease; no matter how well meaning and self-sacrificing they are, they may not be able to deal with the added responsibility. Also, by doing this, you may be creating a co-dependent in your loved one. You may need to talk with a professional to decide this before accepting the help of your loved one.

4. Build your self-esteem by doing something you know you are good at that won't burn your energy away. I write, not only because it comes easily to me, but also by writing I find myself understanding my problems in a non-threatening manner.

5. Keep your life in perspective, and realize there will be some things you must let go of, but then substitute something else. A friend of mine substituted mental aerobics for physical aerobics. She now is considered a mathematical wizard. So what, that you once jogged ten miles, now walk a mile.

Once you supervised dozens of people, now supervise yourself.

6. Determine who you are and what you want. Keep a positive attitude and try to make a success of this new you!

REMEMBER: The childhood story about the engine that huffed and puffed up the hill saying over and over again, "I think I can, I think I can, I know I can!"

7. Promote a baseline of information for self-assessment and personal well being and update this self-assessment regularly.

START with a list of the things you are doing now. Where you live. How you are living. What you eat, your weight, your likes and dislikes in food. Which of these things do you have control over? What would you like to change? This simple list will add much to your aware-ness of your lifestyle. Do it now.[18]

Most childhood disease has been wiped out by the mir-acle of immunization, thus there seems no compelling reason for people to be concerned about preventive health maintenance! A *MYTH* and definitely **Not True**!

Today, most up-to-date health caretakers make it clear that the overall responsibility lies with the individual choices we, each make in our daily living. Health promotion programs emphases a *WELLNESS CONCEPT* that encourages adopting a lifestyle aimed at achieving and maintaining physical men-tal and spiritual well being at home and on the job. We can choose our lifestyles, including: HEALTH, DIET, EDUCA-TION, MARRIAGE, PARENTING, and CAREER just to name a few.

Choosing your new lifestyle takes time. It has taken me over twenty years to accept this reality and to put in place a workable system for myself. It also requires many repetitions. Perfecting your new lifestyle may take even more time. Recall how many attempts it took you to ride a bicycle, to learn to ski, to drive a car. How many attempts will it take you to develop a personal wellness program…a few weeks, possibly months, maybe even years. Don't allow yourself to become discouraged. Did you quit trying to walk when you were two? Nothing worthwhile is achieved in a day![19]

---

18. Reuben, David, M.D.; *Everything You Always Wanted To Know About Nutrition; 1989*
19. Davis, Adelle; *Let's Eat Right To Keep Fit and Let's Get Well and Let's Cook It Right;* New American Library; 1954

I found writing out my excuses for missing part of my wellness plan was important. It identified to me the stumbling blocks I was experiencing, the pitfalls, and most impressively my bad habits. Examples: Driving everywhere instead of walking the extra twenty feet into a store. Nutrition—Eating junk food instead of wholesome grains and vegetables drinking water or juice rather than diet soda. Eating candy for energy, instead of eating a proper meal. Drinking a caffeine soda instead of juice, or water when I was thirsty. A tasty trap definitely, but overall without any long-term benefit. Balance here is all-important[20].

A well lifestyle is an active lifestyle *engaged in living; a winning lifestyle.* Some people are active as a way of avoiding their life; this is not what I'm talking about here. Research proves that people who maintain active lifestyles with a focus on their total well being have fewer health problems than people who live a sedentary life do. The problem for individuals with MS, is not a question of jogging, but one of whether or not they can get out of bed in the morning. A sudden change in an accepted, comfortable lifestyle may do more damage than good. A gradual transition into a more healthy lifestyle is what is needed here, a balance of values in practicing *moderation.*

Each of us has heard the expression, "It's all in the mind." In dealing with a disability this statement seems unfair, and yet is it? For myself, personally, I don't think so. When I was walking like a drunken sailor, I corrected the stumbling gait with energy, time, and a mental exercise. I mimicked a walking person I

20. Hausman, Patricia and Judith Bean Hurley; *The Sugar Blues: Telltale Signs: The Healing Foods, The Ultimate Authority on the Curative Power of Nutrition;* 1989

admired. I made a point to do it every time I walked, whether to the bathroom, or down the street. It was a conscious decision on my part and it worked. All in the mind, you say, the physical evidence points otherwise. Yet, without this mental decision and effort would I be walking normally now? Doubtful, I believe. Each time I stumble and allow my leg to drag it is only because I have forgotten to allow the image to guide me. I forget to use the conscious mind to aid me in my progress. I didn't say it wasn't work.

Each of us experiences pressures and strains in our daily lives. The decisions people make are whether or not to let the anxieties of life take over and control them. Every situation can be perceived as either "stressful or challenging." Some people see life as a series of catastrophes. Those who manage stress the best use terms like challenge, adventure, task at hand, or another positive variation. This attitude is one of coping-rather than being afraid of losing control or being harmed.

Your body can only work with what you put into it. Nutrition is the the most important factors in health care. A good balanced diet will keep your heart healthy and your mind creating. A diet should include the four food groups and be low in saturated fats and cholesterol. There is no need to become a "nuts and twigs" fanatic. It's okay to give in to our vices from time to time. We're talking lifetime habits. Note: You and I need to balance good eating with reasonable flexibility to leave room for socializing and enjoying life. Just keep it all in perspective. This is easier said than done of course—so read "Food and Healing" by Annemarie Colfin for a clearer idea of a balanced diet if you require a thorough understanding of what I'm getting at in this section. Recently some excellent general magazines have appeared that identify individual nutritional elements that are necessary for achieving balance.[21,22]

Athletes, in competition, know that the mental game may be up to 80 percent of their success. A balanced attitude considers the positive and negative outcome of situations. Television, newspapers, unhappy people, and also our own negativity expose us to the negatives. Cutting down on the negative input in our daily lives leaves room for the positive to blossom.[23, 24,25]

How does all this relate to an individual with MS? Doctors and therapists tell us that positive people get sick less often. When they do become ill, they recover more quickly and fully. Is keeping the positive alive each minute of every day too much to ask of individuals with a chronic disease? Or is it another burden added to the constantly growing list? This will be up to the individual again, to decide. But for me, because I needed to be the best that I could be under any circumstance, I adopted my present wellness program.

Only by challenging ourselves can we succeed with this difficult perception—it takes minute by minute work 24 hours a day. It may be difficult to accept at first, but if you try one small step at a time and congratulate yourself for trying to make a life change, then all the other steps will fall into line soon after.

21. *Prevention*; P.O. Box 7585, Red Oak, IA 51591-2585
22. *Longevity*; P.O. Box 3226; Harlan, IA 51593-2406
23. *The Silva Mind Control Method*; Silva, Jose; Pocket Books; 1977
24. *Sick and Tired of Feeling Sick and Tired: Living with Invisible Illness*; Donoghue, Paul J. Ph.D. and Mary E. Siegel, Ph.D.; Norton & Company, New York; 1992
25. *Take Charge of Your Emotional Life: Self-Analysis Day by Day*; Langs, Robert, M.D.; Henry Holt and Company; New York; 1991

Understanding the role food chemicals play in controlling the symptoms of MS helped me to comprehend why a dietary change was absolutely necessary for my well being. Over a decade ago it was discovered that three of the chemical neurotransmitters are manufactured by the body from components in the food we eat. These three chemical neurotransmitters are: DOPAMINE, NOREPINEPHRINE, and SEROTONIN.[26]

Dopamine and Norepinephrine are the alertness chemicals. Research suggests that when the brain is producing dopamine and norepinephrine, changes in mood and behavior take place. We have a tendency to think more quickly, react more rapidly to stimuli, and feel more attentive, motivated, and mentally energetic, heightened brainpower and a feeling of being on a mental roll.

Serotonin is the calming chemical. When the brain is using Serotonin, feelings of stress and tension are eased and the ability to concentrate is enhanced. When your thoughts are going in too many directions an increase of Serotonin will act like a brake, allowing you to filter out distractions and focus. Serotonin will also slow reactions somewhat and may make you feel sluggish or sleepy.

The body from amino acids synthesizes these three neurotransmitters. Amino acids are organic compounds that form the basic components of proteins. The amino acids that are used to make the neurotransmitters are: Tyrosine in Dopamine and Norepinephrine and Tryptophan in Serotonin. Amino

---

26 Wurtman, Judith J. Ph.D. *Managing Your Mind and Mood through Food*. MIT Research Scientist Paper, M.I.T. Chemistry 1990

acids come in twenty types and are found in protein, so if you eat protein you will feel more alert and energized.

Of the twenty amino acids, Tryptophan is the slowest to get into the brain. When you eat a high protein meal, it is digested (the digestion process makes amino acids from protein) and the amino acids are absorbed into your blood steam. Tryptophan attaches tightly to albumin in the blood and continues to circulate while the other amino acids are absorbed the body cells. The energy used by the cells comes from blood sugar. When this is high (after a high carbohydrate meal) the absorbing mechanism for amino acids are energized.

Eating a meal of carbohydrates only boasts blood sugar that energizes brain cell amino acids so more of the albumin bound Tryptophan is transferred to the brain cells. When the amino acids are not present the tryptophan on the albumin can be "seen better" by the brain cells and the energy to take it from the albumin is available. The brain cells then use the tryptophan to make serotonin that calms you.

So how does Serotonin, made from Tryptophan, calm you if it's from protein? Well, of the twenty amino acids, Tryptophan is the slowest to get to the brain. Think of the bloodstream as a freeway with only one entrance into the membrane surrounding the brain. Studies have shown that increases in protein in diet actually decrease the amount of tryptophan in your brain (tests were only done on animals).

The way to get Tryptophan to your brain is by eating carbohydrates—alone. It works like this: When you eat carbohydrates, i.e. pasta, bread, your blood sugar rises and is released from the pancreas. Insulin regulates blood sugar levels, and it also keeps the amino acids (from our food) moving through the bloodstream to join with bone, muscle, and organ cells. Tryptophan will anchor itself to albumin in the blood and keeps on circulating. Now there is more Tryptophan in the blood than the other amino acids (they got, 'dropped off' somewhere) and now Tryptophan can get on the freeway with very little competition. An alert—nature has a built in regulating system—it is impossible to overdose on the amino acids in foods. However, Tyrosine and Tryptophan are sold in bottle form at health food stores and can be taken orally. Taken in this manner the body may become over stimulated thereby producing very harmful side effects, even death.[27]

THE FOLLOWING IS A LIST OF THE
FOUR FOOD GROUPS

Need a copy of the food pyramid ***

The Best Proteins
(Little or no fat)
Shellfish   Fish   Chicken w/o skin   Veal
Very Lean Beef trimmed of visible fat

Second Best Proteins
Low-fat Cottage Cheese Skimmed or Low/fat Milk/Yogurt
Dried Peas and Beans   Lentils   Tofu and other soy-
bean-based foods
FATS
Carbohydrates (simple and complex)
Starches

---

27. Reuben, David, M.D. *Everything You Always Wanted To Know About Nutrition; 1990*

Breads	Crackers/Muffins/Rolls/Bagels	Pasta
Potatoes	Rice	Barley
Kasha	Corn/including tortillas	Cereals

Oatmeal/w/o milk

Sweets (Glucose is only sugar that will produce immediate increase in insulin)

Candy	Cookies	Pie	Cake
Ice Cream	Jams, Jellies	Syrup	Soft Drinks

Chocolate * (see appendix)

Fruit won't activate the insulin so quickly. Processing of fructose to glucose takes the body time, though fructose is the sweetest of the sugars.

Caffeine should be avoided or moderately consumed at all times. Read about side effects below.

If you've surmised FROM this section of the book that I feel that Nutrition is one critical element in making a change in your MS condition, you are correct. It is central to a program of personal wellness no matter the condition you are dealing with now. As a science, nutrition is relatively new. Almost daily new discoveries are being made linking diet to disease, illness and moods. A healthy diet is preventive medicine, especially if you have a predisposition for certain diseases, i.e. high blood pressure, heart disease, diabetes, MS. A healthy diet also will improve your quality of life—giving you more energy, less illness, fewer headaches, less pain. Eating healthy doesn't cost any more and is reasonably simple. All it takes is a change in habits, in your lifestyle today, or in mine.

Ideally our bodies are composed of 17% protein, 13% fat, and 1.5% Carbohydrates, the rest is water. Drinking plenty of water is crucial—don't substitute sodas, tea, coffee, or milk—drink water. Try for at least four, eight oz. glasses a day, 8 if you can handle them. This will wash out of your body many unhealthy chemicals we consume and help you to refrain from overeating.[28]

Food gives energy that is measured by calories. The number of calories isn't so important as what makes up those calories. The number of calories needed is individually determined. We need to be aware of how we feel and react to foods to determine what our bodies need. EXTREMES ARE FOOL-ISH—*Remember, Consuming A Little Of Everything In Moderation Is Much Wiser Than Overdoing Anything That You Consume.* This book will be addressing averages needed by an adult, without allergies only.[29]

PROTEIN: is needed for growth, repair of the tissues and enzyme, hormone, and antibody production. Protein transports substances through the body. Metabolizes into twenty amino acids; Ten of these amino acids are essential i.e. our bodies cannot synthesis them. Sources are: milk products; meat, poultry and fish, legumes; nuts, and tofu.

CARBOHYDRATES: these are needed for energy and fiber. They are metabolized to glucose and stored as glycogen in the liver and muscles and fat cells (adipose tissue). Excess glucose is converted to fat and stored in fat cells. Carbohydrates are necessary to burn fat properly. Carbohydrates are easiest to metabolize and are high in source of many vitamins and minerals. Sources: grains, cereals; vegetables; fruits; sugar.

28. Colfin, Annemarie; *Food and Healing*, Ballentine Books, 1986
29. Wurtman, Judith J. Ph.D. *Managing Your Mind and Mood Through Food, MIT Research Scientist Research Paper*, MIT Chemistry

FAT: needed for energy and to transport fat-soluble vitamins, D, E, A, K. Provides body insulation and protection. Body metabolizes fat into Glycerol and fatty acids and it is stored in the fat tissues in the body. Fat is the food hardest to metabolize. Sources: oils, butter & shortening; cream, whole milk products; fatty meats; poultry skin; nuts; pastries, pies, cakes; fried foods.

VITAMINS: Nearly everyone in America knows what vitamins are, yet hardly any of us know what they do for our bodies. Don't feel dense if you're a member of the majority. I had no idea what vitamins could do for me until I researched out the available material on them. Unfortunately most of the data is still unclear, but I can assure you that taking Vitamin C, A, and the B vitamins will help you fight stress. Lecithin in capsule form is known to help neurological functioning, plus brain activity and coordination. For me SOYA LECITHIN worked wonders and still does to this day. I highly recommend that any person with a neurological disorder begin taking lecithin immediately to help regain normal use of weakened extremities, and general nerve function. Because certain reserves of vitamins and minerals are more rapidly depleted from a body under stress, (whether organic or lifestyle), it is important to replenish those reserves and to understand what each nutrient does to help fight stress symptoms.[30]

30. Reuben, David, M.D. *Everything You Always Wanted To Know About Nutrition, 1989*

Vitamins and Minerals	Purpose
A	Assists in fighting infections including respiratory infection
SOURCE:	green & yellow vegetables, eggs, organ meats.
B1	Assists in fighting fatigue, depression, & confusion. Promotes emotional stability.
SOURCE:	Whole grains, liver, beans, wheat germ, brewer's yeast, green vegetables.
B2	Riboflavin helps nerves.
B3	Pantothenic Acid. Assists in fighting apprehension and insomnia
Pantothenic Acid	Assists in converting fat and sugar to energy. SOURCE: Liver, kidney, and brewers yeast, sunflower seeds, peanuts SOURCE: Yeast, organ meats, fish, nuts, wheat germ, soybeans.
B6 Pyridoxiene	Aids in the metabolism of fat, assists in fighting nausea and dizziness.

SOURCE: Organ meats, whole grains, walnuts, peanuts, wheat germ, bananas, fish, sun-flower seeds.

Niocene

Folic Acid   Fruits & Vegetables

B12   Necessary for the proper function-ing of the immune system and the nervous system.

SOURCE: Yeast, liver, wheatgerm, milk, eggs, meat.

C   Assists in repairing tissue and fighting infections.

SOURCE: Citrus fruits, green pep-per, chili, broccoli, spinach, toma-toes, baked potatoes, strawberries.

Potassium   Assists in fighting fatigue and forming healthy heart muscle.

Source: bananas and potatoes, cit-rus juices.

Calcium   Assists in forming and strength-ening bones and acts as a natural Sedative.

Source: Milk, bone meal, honey, greens, except spinach.

Magnesium Acts as a natural tranquilize and assists in fighting irritability, take with calcium.

Source: nuts, soybeans, green leafy vegetables, snails.

SOYA LECITHIN
SOFTGELS

Found in all cells of the body acts as a emulsifier of fats and aids the nervous system it builds the messages relaying system.

SOURCE: CAPSULES SOFT GELS
(I take 4 a day—every day)
LESS STRESS FAST FOODS
BANANAS (A, B1, B6, C, POTASSIUM)
ALMONDS (B COMPLEX, COPPER, IRON, CALCIUM, PHOSPHORUS)
RAISINS (B1, B6, CALCIUM, POTASSIUM, COPPER)
BROCCOLI ©
SPINACH (A, MAGNESIUM)
WHEAT GERM (B COMPLEX)
SUNFLOWER SEEDS (E, PANTOTHENIC ACID)
MILK AND HONEY (CALCIUM—NATURAL SLEEPING TABLET)

BASIC FOOD GROUPS AND RECOMMENDED DIET

A. BREADS, CEREALS, AND OTHER GRAIN PRODUCTS (WHOLE GRAIN) SERVING SIZE: 1 PIECE OF BREAD; ½ CUP COOKED PASTA, ¾ CUP UNSWEETENED CEREAL OR 1/3 C COOKED RICE

B. FRUITS
SERVING SIZE: 1 PIECE OR ½ C CUT UP; ¾ CUP UNSWEETENED JUICE

C. VEGETABLES (DARK GREEN, DEEP YELLOW, STARCHY, OTHERS)
SERVING SIZE: ½ CUP COOKED OR 1 CUP RAW

D. PROTEIN (LEAN MEATS, EGGS, FISH, POULTRY W/O SKIN, BEANS, NUTS, SEEDS ETC.)
SERVING SIZE: 1 OZ MEAT, FISH, OR POULTRY, ¼ C BEANS.

E. DIARY PRODUCTS: MILK, CHEESE, and YOGURT Low/Fat SERVING SIZE: 1 C MILK, 1 C YOGURT, and 1.5 OZ CHEESE

F. FATS, SWEETS
SERVING SIZE: REMEMBER MODERATION! I WOULDN'T SUGGEST MORE 1/3 CUP OF ANY OF THESE FOR INSTANCE, AND NO OTHER FATS FOR THE DAY.

G. THE ABOVE SUGGESTIONS ARE FOR MAINTAINING YOUR CURRENT WEIGHT. TO DROP WEIGHT EITHER INCREASE ACTIVITY OR DECREASE FOOD INTAKE. I WOULD START WITH FAT! IF YOU'RE NOT EATING

THIS WAY NOW AND START YOU'LL PROBABLY LOSE WEIGHT ANYWAY OR AT LEAST I FEEL A WHOLE LOT BETTER!

SUBSTANCES TO AVOID

A. REFINED SUGAR:
Has no benefit in the human diet, no vitamins, no minerals, no fiber. It's a manmade poison and can be chemically compared to cocaine, both are psychologically addictive, both produce strong physical and emotional effects, both derive from common plant sources.

CHOCOLATE: ALL TYPES—has been found to inhibit neurological functioning.

B. FAT
Anything containing fat should be limited. It is linked to the following diseases. Cancer increases the severity of diabetes, fibrocystic breast disease, gallstones, high blood pressure, obesity, hearing disorders, Meniere's disease.

C. ALCOHOL—BECOMES GLUCOSE AND WHICH BECOMES FAT IN OUR BODIES
Is implicated in the following diseases; anemia—encourages the excretion of B vitamins; cancer link, hiatal hernia, high blood pressure, ulcers.

D. CAFFEINE/COFFEE/TEA/SODAS
Caffeine enters all organs and tissues of the body within a few minutes of ingestion. Ninety percent is metabolized and only 10% is excreted unchanged in the urine.

Caffeine's effects may be subtle and obscured by the multifaceted nature of many chronic disease states.

Some may be thinking; "hey, everybody drinks coffee, tea, or cola and eats chocolate...can it really be all that bad? Understanding some of the side effects of caffeine may be all that is needed for individuals with MS to discontinue consuming anything with caffeine. (I know that if I had been aware of these side effects of caffeine 15-20 years ago I would have prevented several uncomfortable hospital stays and eliminated permanent damage to my neural system).

I will only list the central nervous system effects of caffeine. There are others dealing with the gastrointestinal system, respiratory system, kidneys, urinary system, reproductive, bladder, prostate, thyroid, infections in general, and caffeine has been linked to a predisposition of women to fibrocystic breast disease. Withdrawal symptoms usually cease after two or three days and can include a) headaches, b) drowsiness c) runny nose and nausea d) cotton mouth e) nervousness and irritability f) trembling with a chill g) insomnia h) even depression and an inability to work effectively. These withdrawal symptoms last up to two weeks or a bit more, depending on the level of addiction.

1. Caffine and the effects on nervous system.
    In children, caffeine may cause damage to the brain
    and central nervous system development. A survey
    revealed pregnant women who consume an average of
    193 mg of caffeine a day, or 5 or more cups of coffee a
    day, cause thousands of birth defects.
    Caffeine is a powerful central nervous system stimu-
    lant. Large doses may impact motor function, where
    delicate coordination is required. It increases reac-
    tion to sensory stimuli, but the post stimulation
    "results in fatigue, lethargy, and depression". All
    mental and physical stimulation ceases when con-
    suming more than two cups or two cola's in two
    hours. After two cups coffee, caffeine acts to slow all
    reaction times and impairs thinking ability.
    High doses can produce symptoms indistinguishable
    from anxiety neurosis. Caffeine causes nervousness,
    irritability, muscle tension, and trembling. It can cause
    headaches, shaky hands, and even hallucinations. High
    doses 20 cups or 400 mg of caffeine can cause grand
    malseizure, respiratory failure, and death.
    Caffeine is the principal cause of "restless leg syn-
    drome"This results in insomnia and an uncomfortable
    feeling caused by involuntary movement, (jerking) of
    the legs or hands. It has significant effects on muscle
    contractions relaxing smooth muscles and increasing
    the contraction of skeletal muscles.
    Caffeine may mask mental and physical fatigue. This
    maybe dangerous while driving. It interacts with other

drugs and decreases barbital-induced sleeping time. Caffeine is habit forming and addictive.

Both coffee and tea destroy thiamine (vitamin B1) because of their high caffeine content. Any heavy caffeine user is likely to be deficient in B1, which is crucial to mental health and tranquility. Lack of thiamine causes nervous exhaustion, fatigue, loss of appetite, loss of memory, depression, constipation, inability to concentrate, feeling of inadequacy, lethargy and intense drowsiness.

Caffeine has been known to trigger psychosis, through its action on a set of chemicals in the brain called neurotransmitters. These convey messages across microscopic gaps, called synapses, between nerve cells in the brain and muscles.

What about caffeine-free coffee and soft drinks, you may now ask? A chemical used in making decaffeinated coffee (TCE-tricholoroethylene) has been known to cause liver cancer. The National Cancer Institute also warns against using three possible substitutes for TCE. Replacing a chemical with carcinogenic risk with another chemical of unknown risk may result in a more hazardous alternative. In other words, all the side effects of the chemical used in decaffeinated coffee, tea, etc. are still unknown. Caffeine-free soft drinks and sugar-free soft drinks still have substitutes and chemicals. It is best striving to develop a taste for healthy beverages. Think of how much beverage is consumed during a lifetime! It's the fluid your body uses to trigger every chemical reaction and enzyme activity. If you think a few chemicals in the beverages we drink don't make any difference in how people feel, try putting one percent water in a gas tank and see how well a car runs.

The most obvious question following this lengthy aside on the effects of caffeine drinks and chocolate is, "If I can't drink coffee, tea, alcohol, soft drinks, or even eat chocolate what is left for me?"

Fresh spring water is my first answer. Everyone should drink up to 8-10 glasses of water a day to provide the body with needed fluid. After strenuous exercise on a hot day, nothing quenches thirst like water. I place the juice of a fresh lemon in a cup of hot water finding it a good way to start the day and it also helps me with weight loss.

Next try carbonated spring water (Perrier) plain, lemon, lime, or orange. It can be purchased at any grocery store. It contains no calories, sugar, or chemicals. It is a good, carbonated, refreshing substitute for cola. Next try sugar-free fruit and vegetable juice. A healthy investment could be a vegetable/fruit juicer to produce fresh juice. Nothing tastes better or is healthier for you than freshly juiced fruits and vegetables. Lastly most stores have natural cereal beverages to replace coffee that are very pleasant tasting. Some popular ones are Sipp, Caffix, and Pero. I have become quite creative with my beverages and I know you will to once you have made the commitment to a life without caffeine.

Beverages	Caffeine mg
Decaf Coffee	2
Filter drip coffee	110
Percolated Coffee	85
Dark Chocolate	80
Instant Coffee	65
Leaf Tea	40
Milk Chocolate	35
Cola not decaf	25
Cocoa	15

Note: Coffee from South American beans usually contains about half as much caffeine as African *coffee* beans.

E. SODIUM (salt)

Implicated in the following diseases: high blood pressure, water retention, headaches, and ulcers

F. FOOD STORAGE:

Nutrition wise food storage and preparation is not a science. Home cooking methods used are largely those that have been handed down from generation to generation and date back to the time the science of nutrition was unknown. The nutrients in many foods are either destroyed or thrown away before the food reaches the table. If health is to be gotten from the food we grow and buy, care must be taken in the handling and preparation. Many vitamins are destroyed by oxidation and dissolved in water.[31]

---

31. Colfin, Annemarie, *Food and Healing*, Ballentine, 1986

Not all foods are created equal and milk, labeled low fat can contain more butterfat than buttermilk. Here are some more nutritional surprises that may shock you.

Drinking orange juice with your meals can boost your body's absorption of iron from the plant foods by as much as 400 percent, because vitamin C, abundant in oranges, enhances iron's bioavailability. The body cannot readily absorb this means up to 90 percent of the iron in plants normally. Red and green peppers have almost 1-½ times more vitamin C, than oranges.

Chasing an iron rich dinner with a cup of coffee or tea can reduce your body's absorption of minerals by 40-80 percent. The culprit, apparently, is tannin in tea and coffee, which binds with iron.

Ounce for ounce, cauliflower also has more vitamin C than oranges. In fact, just one cup of cauliflower delivers more than the U.S. RDA daily requirements.

Tofu, a high-protein soybean curd, actually contains more than half its calories in fat unless you get low-fat or non-fat brands. The good news is that, unlike animal protein, tofu is mostly mono- and polyunsaturated fat with no cholesterol.

Not all turkey products are as lean as you may think. While skinned turkey breast has less than 5 percent fat calories, turkey bologna and franks can contain up to 70 percent fat.

Cooked Brussels sprouts, corn, zucchini, pintos, lima beans, raw cauliflower and fresh currants all have as many cholesterol-lowering soluble fibers per half cup as does cooked oatmeal.

Shellfish are generally high in cholesterol but surprisingly low in saturated fat; four large raw shrimp, for example, tip the scale with 152 milligrams of cholesterol; but a scant third of a gram of saturated fat.

Trimming visible fat from meat and skinning poultry can cut the saturated fat content by more than one-half; interestingly, still, it has very little effect on the cholesterol content.

Lastly, a potato has almost double the potassium of a banana.

Rules For Saving Food Value[32]

1. Purchase only the amount of fresh food that you need or that can be kept in refrigeration.

2. Wash all food quickly.

3. Avoid peeling whenever possible

4. Slice, grate, chop, crush foods when they are thoroughly chilled. Prepare before serving or cooking.

5. If foods must be prepared in advance, cover them from air and store in refrigeration.

6. To freshen salads, sprinkle with water and keep in a plastic container.

7. Soak no food unless it is dried (lentils, beans, etc.) and then use only the amount of water that it will absorb.

8. Reheat canned foods in their juice.

---

32. Reuben, David, M.D. *Everything You Always Wanted To Know About Nutrition*; 1989

9. Steam, steam, and steam! If food must be boiled put in water already boiling.

10. Use the shortest cooking methods and heat foods rapidly. Don't over cook! Leave color and a little crunch.

11. Start cooking frozen vegetable before they are thawed.

12. Serve frozen fruits immediately after thawing if they are to be eaten raw.

13. Never Overcook!

14. Don't throw away liquid in which foods have been cooked.

   Keep in a covered jar in the fridge and use for soups!

15. Buy a food juicer and juice vegetable and fruit juices at home.

Also note, please, that recent research and guidelines published by the US government have revised the four food groups. Now we are told to eat more than twice as much from the breads and cereal group as from any other group.[33]

33. Hausman, Patricia and Judith Benn Hurley, *The Sugar Blues: Telltale Sign: The Healing Foods, The Ultimate Authority on the Curative Power of Nutrition*, New York, 1989

Chapter Five

PART 5

CREATIVE VISUALIZATION
HOW TO DO IT—AFFIRMATIONS
BEING, DOING, AND FAITH—
MEDITATIONS

I stumbled onto creative visualization in the early nineteen seventies. A fellow ranger introduced me to Yoga. I so enjoyed the stretching exercises and meditations that when the doctor told me I was a victim of MS, I immediately sought out ways to help myself from inside myself, as Yoga teaches.

I used this unconsciously during my early years of dealing with this disease, and my eyes to watch others walk. At the time I was stumbling, zigzagging across a normal sidewalk and stepping on my feet. In disgust I looked up and saw a woman walking. I watched her until she disappeared, then I tried to mimic her. I failed, but I did not give up. After a few weeks of doing this in my mind every time I walked, I was feeling much stronger, and more balanced. Soon I was walking normally again. Now I know that what I did was creative visualization; then I was just happy with the results.

Later, after a fall and a twisted ankle, I put this principle to work for myself again in a very conscious fashion. Still, it wasn't until 1989 that I even heard the phrase, 'Creative Visualization' and not until 1989 that I read Shakti Gawain's[34] wonderful book, "Creative Visualization[35]". I highly recommend this book to everyone, and especially those seeking a way to help themselves through the power of their mind.

What is creative visualization? Simply put, it is a technique of using your imagination to create what you want in your life. There is nothing new, or strange about this. Normal people use the mind every minute in some way, whether they are conscious of it or not. Everyone uses their creative powers in some way in their daily life. If you cook for yourself or family you combine the ingredients in varying ways from almost every other cook in the world. If you sing, paint, tell stories to your kids, whatever you are doing you most likely use your imagination. Imagination is a human's ability to create an idea or mental picture in the mind. By using creative visualization unconsciously I used my mind to create a clear image of something I wished to manifest, i.e. walking without the MS gait. Then I continued to focus on this idea or picture consciously every time I walked until I achieved what I was visualizing.

Because I was doing this technique by myself I did not get stuck on being judgmental about the process. I accepted it and quickly it became easy for me to walk normally without actually working on keeping the picture in my mind. Because

---

34. Gawain, Shakti, *Creative Visualization*; New World Library, San Rafael, CA. 1978
35. Gawain,Shakti; *Creative Visualization*; New World Library, San Rafael, CA, 1978

the results were immediate and comfortable I have kept the process alive and working without effort.

For those of you who are wondering what I mean by "visualization," I would say don't get stuck on the term "visualization". We all use our imagination constantly. It's impossible not to, so whatever process you find yourself using, seeing clear distinct images, thinking about seeing the goal or process, even feeling an impression, these all work and are all visualization. Just imagine clearly as possible the process and goal and go to work.

There are four basic steps to keep in mind.

1. SET YOUR GOAL.

    Making your goal realistic to your present condition will make it something that you will appreciate when you see the positive, long-term results. My goal was walking again. By watching others, I saw how it was done in the graphic sense. By trying to imitate the movements others made, I set my boundaries.

    I would advise you to set a goal that is easy for you to believe in, one that you can obtain in the very near future. This way you won't have to deal with negative resistance within yourself, and your success will maximize your feeling of success with creative visualizing. Later, as you practice, you will be able to take on more difficult or challenging problems.

2. CREATE A CLEAR PICTURE OR IDEA WITHIN YOUR MIND.

    By creating a specific idea or picture that was based on my goal exactly the way I wanted it now, I found myself proceeding without wasting a lot of time in doubting that this reality could be with me from now on.

My picture was a woman walking normally down a sidewalk at a steady pace. A simple enough image, but difficult for me to achieve as my legs were wobbling like a drunk's. I remember taking deep breaths as I began, closing my eyes, then stepping forward slowly until I took five normal steps! I was elated, then fell flat on my butt the next step. What went wrong? Five steps isn't enough, I learned, to rate my success, not of five steps or of a week of feeling better. Then what is success?

When I could walk a city block without falling I knew I had succeeded. I walked daily at least one mile, always more if I have the time and the energy. Now it is five miles, or even ten. I rate myself in weeks and months instead of days. And a month of feeling stable is a good sign.

3.   FOCUS ON IT OFTEN.

By focusing on your picture or goal often throughout the day and in your meditations you make this new way of thinking an integral part of your life.

I focus on this image-goal in a non-striving manner. I make it a light, airy thought that follows me throughout my day. By doing this I tend not to hinder the imagination, or the creative thought process.

4.   GIVE THE THOUGHT POSITIVE ENERGY.

As I thought about my goal, I thought of the positive benefits walking properly would have for me. By making these strong positive statements to myself, that it was possible, that it would be a reality for me, I short-circuited the negative barriers that could have stood in my way. I saw myself achieving and benefitting from this new independent method of walking. These positive statements are "affirmations." While using these affirmations I succeeded in suspending any doubts or disbelief I had. As the thought became reality I accepted it without feeling guilty or ashamed, just proud of myself for doing something that had made me better.

Most important, for myself, was acknowledging my success with this new process that was totally outside the normal way I had done things before. Celebrating my success came by discussing this dramatic change with others, and writing down in my diary the benefits of visualizing each step before I took it.

Now that I've shown you how I used creative visualization and shared how I made it work for me, you may ask how did I motivate myself to keep this idea alive and working for my benefit? I suppose it is time to clarify my condition there in Medora, North Dakota where my first major attack occurred. I could no longer hold a pencil in my hand, and so I could not write. Writing had been my strength since childhood, and now I could not even make a first grader's line on paper. I was alone, in a strange new area, with my husband working at a new demanding job. I knew no one, and no one knew me. Only with help could I walk to a car, feed myself, or do any of the household chores. I weighed 129 pounds soaking wet. Still I never considered my condition permanent despite what the physician told me, though months went by with little change in my physical symptoms or in the doctor's prognosis. I still believed deep within myself that I could fight back and win.

This could be disheartening, unsettling, and definitely demoralizing, I know, to the healthy world. Instead of brooding on what I had lost though, all I could think about was what I still wanted to do and what I had to do to achieve it.

My husband's support during this crushing time was invaluable. His faith in me was incredible and I knew that whatever stress I was under, his was doubled at this time. I did everything I could think of to make both of our lives calm without bemoaning my apparent losses. Life got easier as the months flowed by, and we each adjusted to the new diet, and the cycle of rest I required. With humor we supported each other and looked to the future rather than to our past. We still do this though at times we forget how important we have been to each other, and we are still together after thirty years of marriage.

I'm not sure what I would have done without the insights offered by relatives, friends and medical care givers. I do know, I would not have lost faith in my values, my principles, or myself. These are a part of the Circle of Health I had going for me to begin with and they each remain as important today as they were then. My belief in the spiritual brought me forward with the certainty that I had within me the power of the Lord.

Another part of this circle is developing communication skills with the important people in your life. Active listening includes reading body language, and repeating what the other individual is saying so that full understanding can be attained. This takes practice and may be awkward but once I started on this road, everything became easier to understand.

AN EXERCISE

How To Do It
Affirmations, Being, Doing, and Faith

Creative visualization is as easy as wishing for something, anything, wonderful to happen. By expecting a miracle and setting your mind on the positive outcome of your dream. Affirming to yourself that your desire is a good thing for yourself. My desire is walking as normally as possible, all the time.

It takes work, conscious work. I didn't say that it was easy to visualize yourself into a new reality beyond the effects of this disease. I said it was easy to visualize yourself there in a subconscious manner.

The first thing that must go is your acceptance of the limitations of your condition. For myself it meant walking normally again rather than like a drunken sailor. If you totally accept that you are wheelchair bound then you will be. If you decide to try for another reality, then you are bound to fall and feel embarrassed at first, but you must remember you are trying for a new image of yourself. It is very much like losing weight when you're fifty pounds overweight. First you must desire to be thinner, therefore you know you must eat less, and only the proper things for your body. You know exercise helps to burn the unwanted calories; therefore you decide to start an exercise program within your daily schedule. This may only mean instead of riding the elevator up 17 flights of stairs you climb upward six flights, then take the elevator up five more then climb six to reach the office on floor number 17. If you take it one step, or one stair, at a time you can succeed. This is all that I mean by exercising. I now walk a mile a day down to my post box and back, then in the evening I ride my stationary bike until I begin to perspire.

I eat a sensible diet, without red meats. I now have a drip tray for micro waving all beef, fish and poultry so that fat is removed from my food. I am careful not to overload on gravy and other sauces. This may sound bland to you, but rest assured I allow myself the luxury of an occasional piece of vegetarian pizza or enchilada. Diet is as much a matter of visualization as exercise is.

To clarify what I mean by my visualization program I highly recommend the book and tape of Shakti Gawain, Creative Visualization[36]. This book is a clear and practical guide for the beginner or even the advanced student of visualization. It offers inspiration and an uplifting message that acts as a companion to the seeker upon the solo journey of discovery. All the book requires is for the reader to have an open mind and heart, plus the desire to improve their way of being.

---

36. *Creative Visualization: Use the Power of Your Imagination to Create What You Want In Your Life*; Gawain, Shakti; New World Library; San Rafael, California; 1978

For me this book opened a world I had never dreamed of experiencing it and it dramatically changed my view of living. I was excited by the exercises, as they challenged my reality of using my illness as a crutch or an excuse not to expand beyond my limits imposed by MS. With the basics of creative visualization I learned to relax fully for the first time in my life. To accept myself for what I am. I learned the difference between just living each moment of my day, and actually being alive within each moment. I learned the difference between just doing things to fill the hours, and doing things with a greater purpose with the others that are striving toward vitality. I learned the difference between having things, allowing and accepting things and people into my life. I learned the difference between comfortably occupying the same space, while achieving a living unit of wholeness, and supporting others without conflict.

To become successful at creative visualization there are three necessary elements that must be within you.

1. Desire. You must have a true desire to achieve what you seek. A strong, clear feeling of purpose. By asking myself what I desired, and finding my answer, which was walking more normally, I centered on my desire and work toward it daily.

2. Belief. The more I believed in my goal and the reality of achieving it, the more certain I was I could attain it. Doubt can not become a factor here. You must believe your goal is possible beyond any outside evidence.

3. Acceptance. I found I needed to accept and have the reality of walking once more. Making sure I was positive I

actually wanted what I was seeking, rather than the sympathy of others.

The clearer my desire, the easier it was to achieve creative visualization of my goal, and the sooner it will work for you, too. Beyond walking once again, I had other goals that I wanted to achieve. One of these was writing this book and sharing with others our chronic condition, methods of helping themselves past the demoralization of this disease. I found that affirmations were not only strengthening but also acted as a clarifying tool in realizing my goal was not paradoxical, or weak. I tell myself often. "I have the intention to create this reality now!" And I go full force forward to make it so.

Now for the techniques to achieve creative visualization: Through experience you will soon find the particular images and techniques that work best for you.

For myself, I start by relaxing, making sure I am in a place that is quiet and unlikely to be disturbed.

I first take deep breaths, closing my eyes, and relax into a deep meditative state. Then I imagine myself walking down a street busy with pedestrian traffic. I see myself calmly stepping forward. It is important to see each step, one at a time, without any hesitation. By trying to get a feeling that my mental image is possible, I experience it as if it is already happening.

I repeat this short, simple exercise often as I walk, alone or in a crowd. When I am tired, I emphasize to myself that now is the time I need visualization the most to make a success of this new image I've created. By being truly open to change I soon find myself walking without difficulty even on the days when I was feeling an MS flare-up. Eventually I found my walking problem improved to the point that now I only occasionally must "see" myself walking to keep this image as a daily reality.

As Ms. Gawain states, it is not necessary to believe in metaphysical or spiritual ideas, though you must be willing to entertain such ideas as possible. It is not necessary to "have faith" in any power beyond yourself.

I've found that the only thing necessary is to have a "desire" to achieve a new way of "being." An open mind allows you to try something in a positive spirit of success.

If you find yourself meeting with success as you attempt to change your reality, then continue to use and develop your skills and broaden your knowledge and experience. An open heart and mind will lead an awakening spirit. By study and work you may find, as I have, that you are exceeding anything you ever dreamed possible.

For me creative visualization is magic in the highest sense of the word. It involves trusting myself and aligning myself with the natural principles that govern the workings of the macrocosm we live in. By learning the grounding principles of the conscious mind, and using the unconscious creativity alive within each spirit I found that stepping beyond the confines of medical reality was possible.

I still have the diagnosed condition of MS and will until I die. At times I still have flare-ups that are disturbing and unsettling. These times I find myself tested to the extreme, requiring that I place my new vision of myself into focus begin working all over again toward my desire. This is an unending challenge. It makes my life exciting, more fulfilling and challenging than ever before.

CHAPTER SIX

THE EAGLES PERSPECTIVE
THE QUEST FOR DIGNITY AND THE SELF
TAKING CHARGE OF YOUR LIFE AND
THOUGHTS

I was fortunate at twenty-five to have had a physician, the first neurologist who diagnosed me, who laid down the reality of the disease MS, and the probable progression of the malady. I remember clearly his stating that stress was a factor and that stress we create in our lives affected the progression of the disease.

He identified for me some factors I could control immediately, i.e., diet, exercise, and attitude. He did not go into detail by saying I should not consider having a family of my own, or children. But he did outline the reality and responsibility of a parent and the child's dependence on its mother or father. The rest I filled in from my experience in dealing with an ill mother, my family's lack of economic advantages, and poor family attitude toward the ill.

I had decided within myself that children were out for me before I was ever diagnosed with this disease, or ever had a symptom. I clearly recalled my childhood with my ill mother and the times I had wanted her to be able to accompany me to school, or to extra curricular activities. How let down I had been when she had to say no and how guilty I felt for placing this burden on her. I discussed this with my husband of four years then. I gave him the option of parting ways during the initial weeks after my diagnoses with MS and waited for him to make a clear decision about our future relationship.

I was fortunate that he loved me then and that he lacked a desire to end our marriage. I quickly accepted his decision. Six months later, when I was well again, I forgot the offer. Though I've thought about it often during our marriage, he still is firm in his commitment. Now, thirty years later, I realize our partnership has been based on communication and respect. The few times we have been at odds is because our communication system failed. Either I did not clarify my condition to him or I overlooked the need to be open and honest about my feelings or self-doubts. There were times when he failed to question me concerning my reaction to things in our daily lives that were acting as stresses beyond my ability to handle[37, 38].

We're still dealing with these issues. Now, though, we have a deeper understanding of the level of communication needed. We both recognize the work that is involved in keeping our relationship a union of two like-minded spirits with mo re in-depth communication required than that of other couples. The last few years has dumped added stress on this relationship and my continued adjustment has put us at odds

37. Tannen, Deborah Ph.D.; *That's Not What I Meant*; Ballentine Books, 1986
38. Tannen, Deborah, *You Just Don't Understand: Women and Men In Conversation*; Ballentine Books; New York, 1990

of remaining together, but our caring spirits are reluctant to give up on our long term relationship.

We now take charge of our thoughts, and actions. The responsibility lies with each of us to question and share our reactions to the various factors that control our daily lives. Together and separately we have accepted the MS condition and live with it, without blaming each other or the universe[39].

Outside professional help may be needed to gain a perspective on this condition. Acupuncture is a positive force in treating the symptoms without resorting to medications that can, and often do, throw the natural body chemistry out of balance. With a one hour treatment, every month or so, I feel revitalized and more in control than before. This is important for the sufferer of MS. Gaining even an ounce of control over circumstances outside your normal realm of control, is heartening and fulfilling[40].

Outside mental support has been mandatory to help me keep everything in perspective and releases me from the shame and guilt that is an entwined part of this condition. Here I finally recognized myself as a co-dependent[41]. I grew up in a home where illness, prescription drugs to the point of addiction, and alcohol were the norm rather than novelty. It has taken me several years and many false starts to gain a level of detachment from that early lifestyle. After dealing with the grief and sense of loss this soul searching brought on, I immediately recognized that not only had it given me a sense of compassion for myself and others, it also validated my thought processes. My husband

39. Tannen, Deborah, Ph.D. *You Just Don't Understand,*William Morrow and Co. New
40. Pelletier, Kenneth R.; *Holistic Medicine*; Delta Book; 1979
41. Beatty, Melody; *Co-Dependent No More*; Doubleday, 1989

also has used counseling services and gained more strength and wholeness through them.

Believe in yourself and open yourself to others. This has been the most important part of my growth. From here, I now know I can go anywhere and survive with dignity. Each day is a blissful occurrence and I enjoy some part of it as fully as I can, even when I'm battling symptoms.

This doesn't mean I've given up my jobs. No way! I still manage a home, a career as a college instructor (part-time), a writer. I volunteer for the National Park Service, dispatch for the Search and Rescue Team, and for many other community committees as well. It is fun, and I no longer have to sit back and fill myself with self-pity. If nothing else, I can act as telephone massager, typist, or resource leader with my various activities. It's fun to develop my skills and see the results of my work. My brain has not stopped operating just because my legs tend to fail me.[42]

By recognizing myself as a volunteer servant to humankind and donating time to only worthwhile organizations I have found self-worth. These efforts fill the void that results from giving up full time employment in the work-a-day world of the uncompromised majority of health professionals.

I make it my duty to write to others who are ill. I talk to groups about wellness and peer counsel individuals who need bolstering and information about sources to gain professional aid, and have frustrations about finding professional help. I have yet to feel bored or drained because of this

---

42. Masters, Robert Ph.D. & Jean Houston, Ph.D.; *Mind Games, The Guide To Inner Space*; Delta Books, 1972

humanitarian effort. Actually, I feel a new self-worth, and confidence, a knowing within, that I'm doing the right thing for others and myself[43].

And I write down my thoughts. When I can't write (which has happened repeatedly in my 20 years with this disease), I tape 90 minute conversations, working through my thoughts and feelings of inadequacy. By doing this I maintain a positive sense of self and keep a continuing record of my progress[44].

You and I, also every other American, are fortunate to be alive in the 1990's. A new law was passed into effect, in the spring of 1991, known as the Americans with Disabilities Act. This is a broad piece of legislation affecting all people within this country. We are all aware that disabled individuals are a blessed minority but this law has finally recognized that at any moment any American may join our group.

ADA covers a huge segment of society—anyone who has a physical or mental impairment that substantially limits a basic life activity such as walking, breathing, performing manual tasks, hearing, seeing, learning, or working. It applies to all, and prohibits discrimination against many whose disabilities are less evident—none of us are made by Mattel and are Barbies or Ken. Inside MS, the National Multiple Sclerosis Society newsletter Vol. 9 No.4, the fall/winter 1991 issue article on ADA gives not only the specific law enacted by Congress but also identifies tips for employees, and tips for employers. Seek additional information assistance from

---

43. Alies, Roger; *You are the Message: Getting What You Want By Being What You Are*; Doubleday, 1989

44. Masters, Robert Ph.D. & Jean Houston Ph.D.; *Listening To The Body, The Psycho physical Way To Health and Awareness*; Delta Books, 1978

groups such as the National Multiple Sclerosis Society (1-800-624-8236) or the local MS chapter in your area; the Job Accommodation Network (1-800-526-7234); or the Development Team, Inc. (301-563-2170) or the internet address: or if your question is unique call 1-800-344-4871.

From equal access, to job discrimination and equality on the job, this forward thinking act at last recognizes the civil rights of the handicapped minority. It is a thankful blessing. Everyone realizes cultural change takes time to occur and that anything that forces change in people's thinking meets with resistance. But at least one of the biggest battles has been won. Now watch the rest of the issues fall into place.

CHAPTER SEVEN

EACH OF US MUST BE WHAT WE CAN BE—LIVING THE LEGACY

By understanding the basic principles I've built my progress on, it should help each of you undertake a program of healthful enlightenment. Each principle now follows in order of my growing understanding and actual experimentation with each. Through these varied steps I've recognized that each day of my life is becoming fuller, more creative, and more in harmony with the world around me, whether it be human, animal, or nature. Being in harmony is the core of every religion and philosophy. Harmony is balance. Recognizing the pitfalls before you stumble into them takes practice, insight, and experience. The most important word here is 'repetition'.

Don't expect to stumble and fall into some of these pits often. But as you lie there, allow your mind to catalog this fall into a new unseen, or unrecognized encumbrance, that next time you can avoid, or circumvent.

Often, I haven't recognized the pitfall until I'd fallen in repeatedly, but after a few times I woke up to the message, no matter how subtle. Not that I won't fall face forward again, but at least now, by outlining my progress in written form, I am able to identify my pathway. I can recognize patterns, habits, and likely booby traps I've either laid for myself, or that are natural unforeseen realities of daily living.

The following themes will act as guideposts to anyone who wants to take a step ahead of the progress of MS and remain master of their fate.

1.   BELIEF

Believe in yourself. Believe you can master the symptoms of this disease on an hourly, daily basis. Even if all this means is that today you will be able to smile, scratch your nose, lift a foot, walk through your home, or down the street. Believe you can do it.

Beliefs generate our thoughts and emotions. You can create your reality with your beliefs. It is important to recognize your beliefs are part of your conscious awareness also your subconscious reality. You accept them as facts…therefore accept, as fact that you are still the same person you were before you were struck with this disease. If you were graceful and full of fun, you still are. If you were a klutz from the age of one, you most probably will remain one, but now with an adult mentality to back you up and I hope a good sense of humor.

Believe you can lift your feet and support your weight. Believe you can move gracefully, though the reality might be only the limping gait of the handicapped, or more properly the physically challenged. By believing you are doing this with decorum for yourself, you make each stride one of celebration. Each day push yourself a little further until you've attained your goal.

Trust that you can make the difference. Trusting in you is hard work and requires lots of practice but it will pay off. Trust your own mind, your own awareness of your bodies needs and reactions. Especially when dealing with medications. You alone know how you feel, what makes you feel good, what makes you feel bad, and even worse what makes you sicker. Trust that inner voice within you and you will find that change will be inevitable.

Never give up, never allow embarrassment to stall you. Remember, you are doing more than the average soul on this planet, and that takes guts, faith, and appreciation from yourself, if from no one else. You will know when you've gone far enough. Don't exhaust yourself, but continue to make steady progress for as long as you are able, every day of your life.

Beliefs are the basis of everything in our lives. True, it is easy to recognize your political, religious, and professional beliefs, but I'm now talking about your 'core' beliefs—who and what you are; your weight, your height, your health, your relationship with yourself, others, your career, your passions, everything central to your existence.

There is a universal law that states: "You will always live up to your self-image." Therefore, make your self-image graceful, charming, funny, and lighthearted and the world will see you as such. They will admire your courage, your fortitude, and your self-confidence despite the obstacles placed in your path.

I believed that first neurologist when he said that if I made the basic changes in my life, i.e. diet, exercise, nutrition, and reduced the stresses in my day to day routine I could be as healthy as I ever was before, possibly more so. That with time and diligence and belief in myself I would be walking again without evidence of the MS gait. Six months after the diagnoses I made it. Six months later I doubted the evidence of the winter before, and eight months later I was down again with a full blown attack, most likely because I forgot the necessary ingredients to maintain my health.

What I realized, almost too late, was that I had made a serious error in judgment.

First, I had assumed the doctors must be wrong, and second I had made the faulty assumption that if I went back to my normal routine, I would be okay.

I paid for it, but it took me at least six soul searching years, several hospital stays, and many emotional outbursts to accept the facts before me and make the permanent changes my condition required.

The actions required of me were: to realize my physical and psychological limitations and self-imposed beliefs. To admit these limiting beliefs and accept them as real. To make a determined effort to create permanent change. The next step was to rise above the effects of restrictive thinking and to become clear about my intent and make change a daily part of my life. The next step was understanding exactly what I wanted; why I wanted it, and what I was willing to do to get it.

I decided on the spot that I did not want to be considered an invalid by anyone. But I look like an invalid, a voice said within me, when I stumbled, when I walked. 'Why did it bother me what other people thought?' I thought next. Because I have a reputation to think about, a life, a job that is often in the public view and a husband who is proud of me. I wondered, 'What would I be willing to do to rise above this restricted view of myself'. I knew that exercise, (the proper exercise), would strengthen my weak muscles, but the disease would only allow me to go so far. Okay then, I vowed to begin the right exercises that day and continue them until I died. This alone made me' feel better, more self-confident, more in charge. It put me in control of a disease that had taken away my control. It changed my restrictive thinking about my condition—to something positive. It was a challenge.

In effect I finally accepted personal responsibility for my life and health. I looked inside for possible causes and cures; when I did, dealing with the MS condition became a lot easier.

Next, I decided to be *honest* with those closest to me and explain my condition to them. This was not to gain their sympathy, but their understanding of my fluctuating emotions and my inability to eat the foods they and I had loved for a lifetime. To understand my need to reduce my stress and take only jobs that I knew I could handle, was very necessary for me. These were jobs under conditions that would be positive and healthy for me. I had to refocus my attention and priorities.

This was a stumbling point for me. I had always wanted to be tops in the medical field from adolescence on, now I had to remove myself from this highly emotional, stressful occupation. I did so, but my talents were so structured to being a leader it irked me to be just a sideline observer.

I stepped back and hid for years. Then like a flash of light one evening it dawned on me that I could remain involved in the medical realm by writing about the positive aspects of this disease vs. the seemingly overwhelming restrictions.

2.   BLAMING AND VICTIMS

Initially I did not consciously blame anyone for my condition. Instead I was surprised. I mean I had worked for years in the health field. I was a nurse, an EMT, and I had always thought that my lifestyle was good, not excellent, but very good when compared to others I saw. I never used illegal drugs or alcohol. But, I had never thought about a disease without a cure before this—regarding myself, and to have contracted one stumped me for at least a year. I did follow the advice of the first neurologist and quickly saw positive progress and ignored the rest of his advice.

After my third attack I suddenly found myself blaming the Park Service lifestyle for my condition. The stress of isolation, the heat, and the uncertainties were beginning to tell on me. This period was the most difficult for my husband and me to deal with. I quit my NPS job, blaming the high level stress for a relapse in my condition. Actually, it was a combination of factors.

One factor was the heat, another was my disgust that I could not control my emotions, another was a lack of a support group (even a book that might have been an ally), and last was the stress of my work and my husband's career. This included for me doing payroll for 50 people, arranging travel for the same, budget, typing, etc. where I was the only administrative employee. Just dealing with individuals who were at odds with my values, principles, and goals would have been enough for the normal healthy person, but soon I could not see the daylight. My spouse is a law enforcement Park Ranger with management and supervisory responsibility. Mix in my former poor diet, high caffeine intake, and the isolation of our work location, also the constant uncertainties of his work, I broke[45]. In other words, I suddenly burned out and had to escape before I could realize that what I needed most was to relax and find something to enjoy in each day.

I needed to learn to laugh at myself, enjoy my new condition and grow with it, not to resist it at every opportunity or hold 'someone' responsible for my new health and not to even hold myself responsible for fate. I learned to express my feelings openly in a non-belligerent way, and to listen carefully to what other people were saying to me. Slowly I learned to accept those things I could not change.

45. Sheehy, Gail; *Passages; Predictable Crises of Adult Life*, Bantam Books, New York, 1976

It's easier to be a victim and blame others for our condition and circumstances than to take responsibility for our own life. We are each on this earth to learn. An illness is only one test to judge our level of awareness. I believe this last statement completely. For as long as we are learning, we are actively responsible for ourselves.

There is no one to blame when one looks at the situation from this perspective. From a human potential perspective, blame is self-pity. Self-pity is negative programming of your subconscious mind, so it is doubly destructive. Get rid of it.

By realizing the futility of blame I found I was the only one harmed by this illusion. Instead, by recognizing that the disease MS is a test of my fortitude, my courage, and my ability to make a positive statement in others lives, I've overcome most of the stigma attached to this illness.

3.   THE NEGATIVE PAYOFFS OF MS

Recognizing the payoff of being an invalid was important to me. If you are invalid, others do things for you that you either feel incapable of handling, or are too lazy to manage alone. (NOTE: I'm not talking to those individuals who have been bedridden or are no longer capable of handling even the basic needs of daily life, but those of us who find self-pity a way out of working toward living normally.) By allowing others to think you are incapable of handling things, you will receive attention. This is often negative attention, but at least you believe now you are important in the significant other's life—you make a difference.

The main problem that I see in this scenario is that by doing the act "of being unable to do the most simple thing" I lost my self-esteem, my self-confidence, and I was immediately overloaded with self-doubts, and self-pity. The payoff was high indeed, especially when I realized I had lost the understanding and respect of those closest to me.

By analyzing the payoff in this way I felt an electric shock of disgust and sudden awareness. All I had been doing was using self-pity in its most negative fashion. Releasing myself from this, took a reversal of values, and a serious concentration to know the positive things I could do for myself. It has taken years to gain perspective and distance from the situation of both self-blame and MS.

I learned to use creative visualization to get this distance. I placed myself in a video camera and raced the film backward to the point when I was first diagnosed, then rapidly ran it forward through all the events of my attacks and days just proceeding them, then quickly to the end. This rapid view perspective helped me to see my habits, and excuses in a new light. It has helped me to maintain balance and harmony, and to subtract those personality traits that were dead ends. On top of this it was fun to watch everyone in my life running backward or forwards to my whim.

What follows is a baseline of steps I followed to balance myself.

1. I sought professional guidance. Both mental and physical. The emotional guidance aided me in gaining perspective of the situation, the causes and the realities of the disease, and the progress I should be able to make on my own. At most it helped me with inter-personal relationships, guilt that our society seems content to heap on the physically challenged.

   The physical guidance I received was learning what types of exercises were best for me, and how often I should pursue them and to what point. Exhaustion is bad, but thirty minutes a day, three times a week is excellent since you raise the pulse and make exercise a habit. I also, began to learn more about nutrition and the pros and cons of addictive behavior. It has made the difference in weight control, headaches, and mood swings for me.

2. I searched and found alternative caretaking methods: i.e. acupuncturists, nutritionalists, bio-feed back training, and meditation either by myself or with an organized group or a support group of my own making.

3. I paid attention to my diet, and my general health at all times. Right now I'm ten pounds over weight, but at forty-eight I'm working on losing some of it.

4. No more pity parties, in silence when I'm alone or while in public. Instead I do something I enjoy when this type of mood overwhelms me; from reading, to writing, to walking, to just daydreaming, listening to good music, or talking to positive people.

5. I work on concentrating on my abilities rather than my disabilities on a daily basis.

6. I have learned to take one day at a time. The nature of MS poses uncertainties about the future and it is more effective to direct your energy toward solving today's problems rather than worrying about tomorrow's.

7. adjusted my goals to realistic levels so that I could reach them. This meant compromising my activity levels not my principles.

8. In doing all of the above I found I had enlarged my scope of values; attaching importance to qualities other than physical prowess.

9. I have learned to measure my successes by what it is possible for me to accomplish, not by what others accomplish.

10. While I avoid dwelling on my problems, I have found it is important to express my feelings and concerns to appropriate people (spouse, family, close friends, or a professional!).

    Anytime I keep them bottled up inside it only leads to an "explosion" when they do come out.

11. I keep as active as I can within limits imposed by my current MS symptoms. By limiting my activities it does not mean that I withdraw from the world or my social contacts.

12. I remember that I must accept myself, before I can expect others to accept me.

MASKS OR ACTS WE HIDE BEHIND

Halloween is fun! Dressing up and pretending to be someone you aren't, remaining anonymous and carefree makes the world seem worry free. Unfortunately, this special day lasts only twenty-four hours, or does it?

For people who have a chronic illness the mask we put on for others is alive and well every hour of every day. This mask blinds us to the obvious. We may lie and say we have the flu when we are tired or frightened, or that we broke our ankle when we limp. But any observer with half a brain knows there is something beyond the lie. There is another reason for our stumbling behavior or our mistakes. Eventually the mask is torn from us by the reality of a lost job, a lost love, or our own under-confidence.

Mask replacements are difficult. The mask acts as a barrier of over-protection from reality. This means if you don't recognize you're hiding and over-compensating, then you won't admit even wearing a mask. It will take another's eyes and insights to wake you up. Therefore, trust your counselors, your support group. Listen and take the advice offered.

Recognizing the masks I hid behind was painful. I needed the mask to cover up the real me, I thought, because I felt the real me was not adequate, impressive enough, kind enough, or loving enough. So by wearing my mask I pretended to be more than I was. I learned masks are fear disguised. There is no way to repress who you really are. When we try, eventually it will show up in an ulcer, a divorce, a heart attack, cancer, or an incurable disease like MS.

By understanding why I wore the mask, I was able to deal with my restrictive thinking. I learned what the fear was behind it. Decide if the reason you wear your mask is valid to your life anymore. Analyze the cost of wearing your mask. How has repression manifested itself in your life? Realize that all you must do to remove the mask is to be direct and honest in your communication with others and most importantly with yourself.

You, and you alone, will know if this advice is sound. Of course it is normal to resist, to deny, to grow angry: but the degree of your anger is only a reflection of the value of the advice. Mull over the advice and take a long, hard objective look at yourself, then ask yourself whom you're fooling with your lie.

When I did this I laughed aloud at the ridiculous irony I had created around myself. I had fooled myself by saying that no one was interested enough to pay attention to what I was doing. The shock of awareness I received, came from a child. Like all children they often recognize what we, adults feel is beyond their comprehension. If only as adults we could maintain the innocence of non-judgement.

CHAPTER EIGHT

MAY THE FORCE BE WITH YOU
MAKING THE COMMITMENT

There are three ways to make a change in any human being or, more importantly, in yourself.

1. Add something to your life; people, things, environment, awareness, programming, challenge etc.
2. Subtract something from your life.
3. Be yourself. Accepting yourself for what you are. This is almost metaphysical in many ways but the most important of the three. And for me the most eye-opening[46].

By now you should have identified for yourself your values and goals. Recognizing those that are incompatible with a healthy lifestyle. This one is probably the hardest for a lay person like myself to write about. I can only look at my goals and values in relating this to the majority.

I wanted to be a physician from an early age. I went to work in a hospital at the ripe age of thirteen as a Candy Stripper, at 15 as a nurse's aid, a year later as an LPN, and a year after that I was studying for my R.N. I still was not out of high school. I

---

46. Tannen, Deborah; *You Just Don't Understand*; Ballantine Books, New York, NY, 1990

sacrificed my adolescence for a dream. Nothing wrong with that, I thought, it was my future.

I was focused and good at what I did. I was encouraged by others, and I glibly lied about my age so that there was no question that I was old enough to be where I was, doing what I was doing. Very few ever asked how old I was, attesting to my apparent maturity and strength of character. I was on my way, until one day I had a sincere talk with a physician I respected at the hospital where I worked. This M.D. laid down the realities for me and clarified my goal.

He pinpointed the dedication becoming a physician would require, the long hours, the lack of sleep, the toll on family life and loved ones, the years of study, the hardship of becoming established in a field that was, and remains highly competitive. There would be constant changes, minute by minute uncertainties, life and death decisions based on nothing more than fate. It was a very sobering discussion for a sixteen-year-old but he promised that if I could manage four years of college and be accepted to a pre-med program, then he would help pay my way through medical school. Wow! And Wow again!

I strived harder to meet this goal, and in my third year of college I suddenly recognized what the M.D. had meant by saying it would take super-human dedication, forsaking all others for the Hippocratic Oath to succeed. I stalled.

Oh, I was still certain I could make the grade, but giving up all my enjoyments, limited though they were at the time, hurt more than I wanted to admit, or could accept. Instead I replaced my goals with my new husband's goals. Quickly proving that I was a valuable member of my new avocation, in a way just as stressful, as my former pursuits, of course it has taken me years to see the similarities, but they are there, and always will be whenever I throw myself full force into a new endeavor.

Another pitfall! This example is graphic and central to my life. Whatever I do I tend to throw my whole being into the raging current. When, within the current I turn around 360 degrees and swim against the current, again fooling myself by thinking I'm swimming in a different direction and then it overwhelms me. It's not the goals that are incompatible with my personality or this disease, it is my struggle to keep afloat. This is a sure sign of a compulsive obsessive personality who strives for perfection. When my goal was not achieved for whatever reason, I felt guilt, self-defeat, lack of confidence, and low self-esteem.

Amazingly it took me seventeen years to realize this, and it will most likely take me another seventeen to put into practice a complete wellness program. What did I say about pit-falls, and shortsightedness and repetition? This last statement is facetious to a degree. I began a nutritional program of vitamins, no red meats, and drinking plenty of water immediately after first being diagnosed. I have consistently walked daily, a mile at least three times a week in good weather, supplementing that with swimming in an outdoor pool as often as possible.

I am constantly working on the stresses in my life by working only part-time at jobs I enjoy. Attending and teaching classes is now my first love, in other words, gaining knowledge and sharing it. I do this best when I write, though I still consider myself a novice, after thirty years of trial and error, with a variety of published books, I know this is what I should be doing.

Also, I make a point to say I've enjoyed each day in some way and usually can identify the feeling later when I'm tired and need revitalization. This is part of my therapy, also a necessary part of being positive and in control of my life and thoughts. Dr. Bernie Siegel's[47] books are another source that I've read and digested, realizing a double dose of wit can build confidence while making the commitment to the mind-body connection.

The National Multiple Sclerosis Society with its 150+ local chapters and branches throughout the country, offers a variety of services that are designed to provide practical assistance, emotional support, and accurate information to people with MS and their families.

Services vary from chapter to chapter due to the special needs of local communities and the resources available. Many chapters, however, offer:
—Comprehensive updated literature
—Information about medical and financial aid
—Counseling
—Medical and self-help equipment
—Newsletters
—Medical symposiums
—Home care training

47. Siegel, Bernie S., M.D.; *Love Medicine & Miracles: Lessons Learned About Self-Healing from a Surgeon's Experience with Exceptional Patients*; Harper & Row Publishers, New York; 1986

Contact the National Society's chapter nearest to your home for any further questions you may have. See Appendix A for addresses and phone numbers of the national chapter.

Research is ongoing, and new treatments are being developed constantly. Keep abreast of the latest by reading and consulting your doctor. Two of the newest western treatments for relapsing-remitting MS exacerbations are Beta-seron (Interferon beta-1b) and Copolymer-1 (Capaxone), Avonix, and Novantrone. All medications are self-injected except Nactune that must be IV injected while under the eye of a physician; the cost is beyond most non-insured individual's ability to pay. The sideeffects of these chemicals are still being studied and the records of remissions are in long-term study at this point. My own personal reaction to Beta-Interferon was one of antaflatic shock, worse than a bee sting, my legs went into rigidity and my blood pressure shot up to over 190/140. This allergic reaction is uncommon, but others have had reactions to these medications. Just be aware and make sure your personal physician remains involved at all stages of treatment.

Another developing therapy is T-Cell replacement. Each of us has T-Cells, which are responsible for making new bone marrow, to skin. By removing an individual's T-Cells then radiating them and reinserting them into the host's body the memory of MS is alleviated. This incredible procedure is still in the experimental stages in 1998 but by the turn of the century may be a common practice for all MS sufferers.

Natural treatments recently developed have also shown positive results. These treatments are thousands of dollars less expensive and the side effects are minimal or non-existent. PECA, or EAP, was developed by the Koehler Company and doctor Robert C. Atkins, M.D. from Germany. The mineral supplement, known as PECA or EAP, is a natural calcium substance also known as colamine phosphate. It has a high affinity to the intracellular space in humans. Calcium EAP is not a drug. It's part mineral (calcium) and part phosphatdyl ethanolamine, a chemical found in the protective covering of nerve cells. EAP carries calcium to the nerve cells where it prevents the electricity involved in nerve transmissions from dissipating. Dr. Atkins has found it useful in all autoimmune disease; lupus, rheumatoid arthritis, Crohn's disease or colitis, Type I diabetes and more. The release of calcium from CA-EAP takes place slowly so that a continuous and steady efficacy can be assured. In 1987 a study of the use of this compound in its injectable form, by 151 Americans with MS, showed the disease's progression was reversed in 63% of the subjects. Nineteen percent of the test subjects stabilized their condition with the substance, and only 18 percent suffered further nervous system deterioration. Overall few if any side effects were reported; something that Beta-Interferon or any other drug cannot claim. Unfortunately, the injectable form has been subject to import seizures by the Food and Drug Administration, calcium EAP still is being obtained and used by thousands of MS sufferers in its pill form; call: 1-206-424-6025 the Koehler Company to obtain product news and descriptions of all their other products that may aid other conditions. [48,49]

---

48. Atkins, Robert C., Dr.; Multiple Sclerosis; Complimentary Approach Succeeds Where Conventional Medicine Fails; Vitamin Cottage Health Hotline; August 1994.
49. Koehler Company, P.O. Box 1508, Mt. Vernon, Washington, 98278; Phone 206-424-6025 or Fax (206) N424-6029

Remember that MS does create some permanent damage and even if a new vaccine is developed, what was lost is rarely returned unless new training and perceptions are developed within the individual. Therefore, seek out alternatives.

Remember each day starts with a new challenge, no matter where you are.

Always keep in mind that you are only one human. You are not guilty of anything. But it is your responsibility to try to find ways to help yourself and make permanent change a real part of your life. Self-responsibility is part of why we were born human I believe. The ability to make choices for ourselves allows us the privilege of health. And life is difficult at best, but with a conscious effort it can be so much better.

CHAPTER NINE

CONCLUSION:
A Successful Life Is My Work of Art

I think of myself as a writer. A writer is an artist who manipulates words instead of paint. Writing is an intricate mosaic combining desire, apprenticeship, blunders, and finally success. Living awake is even more complex and mysterious.

If living is so complicated, then why should I be surprised by the different challenges it presents to me daily, even from minute to minute? Every moment is a moment of creation for me, and the infinite possibilities are fantastic and a challenge.

I may do things the way I've always done them, or I can seek out alternatives and try something new and possibly more rewarding. Each moment presents a new opportunity and a new decision. It is wonderful to have the chance to try the possibilities before me despite my Multiple Sclerosis with creative excitement.

I believe I'm on this earth for a reason and that reason gives my life a mission. By writing I know I can touch and change others and grow within myself. Through the written word I know I am worthwhile. I know you are too.

I found my kernel of power[50] as a child by writing poetry and watching as it was printed and accepted by adults as a solid

---

50. Jamison, Kaleel; *The Nibble Theory, and the Kernel of Power*, Paulist Press, New York, 1984

historical picture of New Mexico. This created my self-worth, non-dependent upon my age. I was only eleven at the time.

You too, have a kernel of power. Look inside and find it. If it is hard to find this kernel it may be because we disguise it by left-brained thinking. Often we identify our skills rather than our personal strengths. It is the unique strengths within yourself that I'm addressing here.

I am asking you to look inside and identify what is uniquely yourself. Like snowflakes we are all related, yet completely different. Once you find this kernel you will find it much easier to remain centered through all life's stresses. Achieving self-understanding will link you to your health, nutrition, exercise, and the importance of believing in yourself. This search may cause you some distress and tears, but that only makes you, human, nothing less. Everyone who undertakes this quest is touched in their center, the emotional pinnacle of their core.

Your unique qualities are there, just like the sun that hides behind stormy clouds. They are there every minute of every day, but until you recognize them, they remain in the unconscious part of your being.

Life is for living, for celebrating. I admire life; its toughness and vigor to remain alive, its recurrence each spring, the challenges it endures, and its consistency despite death, despite unconsciousness, despite desire, despite despair; its spiritual honesty.

I'm persistent, that is part of my core. Also I've acknowledged that I am a risk-taker. I'm consistent with my compassion, my ideals, and my need to become a more whole person by helping others. I am excited about learning something about everything and watching the light go on in others' eyes as they wake up to the glory of more knowledge. I am a seeker: a questioner. I want to grow as much as I can, but I believe I'm here to help others grow as much as they can.

I'm talking about self-acceptance no matter the physical limitations. Put aside your self-criticism long enough to find your strengths[51].

Once they are found you'll find your unique reason for being. Don't be concerned if this search takes you days, weeks, or years. Take time to listen—and to sense what is happening to yourself. It takes practice—understanding—and patience. Remember the lifetime search by the Knights of the Round Table for goodness and honor. Think of yourself as a Knight on an internal pursuit of strength, growth, and risk as I do. It makes the quest fun. An adventure we can take all by ourselves.

Remember a new attitude involves keeping the stress in your life under control. A daily dose of self-assessment, evaluating how I am handling stress in my life, keeps me alert to the pit falls. The basic attitude changes I've made a part of my day include:

* Keeping the pleasant aspects of my life in mind.
* Not dwelling on my failures
* Setting worthy goals for myself, not to waste time and effort on the trivial.
* No procrastinating, this only creates stress.
* Striving for self-improvement, but not perfection; knowing I no longer have to prove myself to be a worthwhile person.

---

51. McNally, David; *Evan Eagles Need A Push: Learning To Soar In A Changing World*; Transform Press; 1990

* Looking deep within to find my spiritual consecutiveness to all of nature and the world and God.
  * Seek out challenges and dare to risk a change in my life.
  * I've taken control.

Now that I understand the condition as identified by Mr. Cayce, (see treatment section) I have also begun research on not only the spiritual body but what is meant by the magnetic body. This research has led me to reexamine the need for such chemical aids as Betaseron and Co-Polymer-1 and alternatives and natural supplements known as EAP or PECA, magnets, the Rife machine, massage and the value of streching the body on an houly basis.

I invite each of you to join me in the ever-changing mosaic of life and feel the beauty that surrounds us. The ever-changing art form of living each day to its fullest, no matter the body's condition. This attitude adjustment will make a dramatic and positive change in your perspective if nothing else. It will make you a freer person with joy a part of your internal personality because at last you understand yourself. This inner personality must be seen and appreciated by those around you. It makes your life, and theirs, easier to accept and deal with.

Smile and say to yourself, as I do each day, "It's a magnificent day to be alive, breathing and using my mind and enjoying everything around me, even my pain."

NOTE:

***

INSERT LATEST INFORMATION ON: Up Date information on each of these:

New Western Drug Therapies/Treatments—Betaseron, Co-Polymer- One, Copaxone and Nautrone

Treatments, Tomorrow's Medicine Today, Dr. Julian Whitaker & Dr. Williams Alternatives

MS Enzyme Therapy: The Turning Point

MS Focus Magazine of the Multiple Sclerosis Foundation, Inc.

Nikken Magnetic Therapy

The Enchanter, MS National MS Society Magazine, Rio Grande Chapter

Spontaneous Remission: The Spectrum of Self-Repair. Caryle Hirishberg

Immune Power Personality, Henry Dreher

Honeybee Healing (AKA Apitherapy) Bee Venom King of America, Charles Mraz

Rife Tool

T-Cell Therapy

APPENDIX A—SERVICES

Multiple Sclerosis Chapter Services vary from chapter to chapter due to the special needs of local communities and the resources available. Many chapters, however, offer:

—Comprehensive updated literature
—Information about medical and financial aid
—Counseling
—Medical and self-help equipment
—Newsletters
—Medical symposia
—Home care training

Contact the National Society's chapter nearest to your home for any further questions you may have. STAY ABREAST OF THE LATEST THEORIES AND TREATMENTS THROUGH YOUR CHAPTER OFFICE—THEY DO.

Multiple Sclerosis Society
New Mexico Chapter
2608 Monroe NE
Albuquerque, NM 87110
(505)-888-4418

Multiple Sclerosis Society
National Office
205 East 42nd St.
New York, NY 10017
(212)-986-3240

World Wide Web address: http://www.nmss.org

MS Questions that are unique: 1-800-344-4867

National   Health   Information   Clearing   House
1-800-336-4797
National Library of Medicine 1-800-638-8480
Mental Health Hotline: 1-800-433-5959
Job Raising Program for People with MS: 1-301-563-2170

INFORMATION ABOUT ADA, (AMERICANS WITH
DISABILITY ACT) CAN BE FOUND AT ANY LOCAL
LIBRARY—JUST ASK
IFORMATION ABOUT EPA OR PECA: KOEHLER COM-
PANY, PO BOX 1508, MT. VERNON, WASHINGTON 98273
TELEPHONE: (206) 424-6025 OR FAX (206) 424-6029.

Appendix B—Stress Tables

Directions: Review the changes in your life over the past few months. Think about each question for about 30 seconds. Rate each. Remember: this is only a reduced version of the test.

1 = No Change 2=Little Change 3=Moderate Change

4=Considerable Change 5=Major Change

_____ Do you tire more easily?

_____ Feel fatigued rather than energetic?

_____ Are you working harder and harder and accomplishing less?

_____ Are you increasingly cynical and disenchanted?

_____ Are you often invaded by a sadness you cannot explain?

_____ Are you forgetting appointments, deadlines, personal items?

_____ Are you increasingly irritable? Short-tempered?

_____ Are you often disappointed in people around you?

_____ Are you seeing close friends and family less?

_____ Are you too busy to do even personal routine things?

_____ Are you suffering from physical complaints (aches, pains)?

_____ Do you feel disoriented when the activity of the day halts?

_____ Is joy elusive?

_____ Are you unable to laugh at a joke about yourself?

_____ Does sex seem like more trouble than it is worth?

_____ Do you have very little to say to people?
_____ Have you suffered an immediate family death recently?
_____ Have you had job difficulties in the past six months?

_____ TOTAL

SCORING: 0-25 You are doing fine
26-35 There are a few things you should watch
36-50 You are a candidate for cumulative stress
51-65 You are well into cumulative stress
65- + You are in danger. Your physical and mental health are threatened.

UPDATED 1990'S STRESS SCALE
BY: PSYCHOLOGIST GEORGIA WITKIN

LIFE EVENT	MEAN VALUE
DEATH OF SPOUSE	97
DISABLED CHILD	97
SINGLE PARENTING	96
DIVORCE	91
REMARRIAGE	89
DEPRESSION	89
CHILD'S ILLNESS	87
INFERTILITY	87
SPOUSE'S ILLNESS	87

SPOUSE'S PROMISCUITY   87
MARRIAGE   85
DEATH OF CLOSE FAMILY MEMBER   84
CRIME VICTIMIZATION   84
FIRED AT WORK   83
HUSBANDS RETIREMENT   82
PARENTING PARENTS   81
RAISING TEENS   80
CHEMICAL DEPENDENCY   80
PREGNANCY   78
MARITAL SEPARATION   78
PARENTS ILLNESS   78
SINGLEHOOD   77
ADOPTION   74
JAIL TERM   72
PERSONAL INJURY OR ILLNESS   68
DEATH OF CLOSE FRIEND   68
RETIREMENT   68
CHILDREN RETURNING HOME TO LIVE   61
CHANGE OF FINANCIAL STATUS   61
SPOUSE BEGINS OR STOPS WORK   58
OWN RETIREMENT   58
MARITAL RECONCILIATION   57
COMMUTING   57
CHRISTMAS   56
CHANGE IN HEALTH OF A FAMILY MEMBER   56
FORECLOSURE OF MORTGAGE OR LOAN   55
SEX DIFFICULTIES   53
ADDITION OF NEW FAMILY MEMBER   56
CHANGE TO DIFFERENT LINE OF WORK   51

BUSINESS ADJUSTMENT	50
MORTGAGE OVER 100,000	48
CHANGE IN RESIDENCE	47
CHANGE IN NUMBER OF ARGUMENTS WITH SPOUSE	46
CHANGE IN RESPONSIBILITIES AT WORK	46
BEGIN OR END SCHOOL	45
TROUBLE WITH BOSS—CO WORKERS	45
VACATION	43
CHANGE IN LIVING CONDITIONS	42
CHILDREN LEAVING HOME	41
OUTSTANDING PERSONAL ACHIEVEMENT	38
CHANGE IN WORK HOURS OR CONDITIONS	36
CHANGE IN SCHOOL	36
MORTGAGE OR LOAN LESS THAN $10,000	27
CHANGE IN SLEEPING HABITS	27
CHANGE IN RECREATION	26
CHANGE IN CHURCH ACTIVITIES	26
CHANGE IN FAMILY GET TOGETHERNESS	15

TOTAL _____

RATING SCALE: ADD UP POINTS OF EVENTS YOU'VE EXPERIENCED IN THE PAST YEAR. YOU CAN DETERMINE WHETHER YOU ARE AT INCREASED RISK OF ILLNESS OR SERIOUS DEPRESSION IF YOUR SCORE IS MORE THAN 400 POINTS? BEWARE AND TAKE ACTION.

STRESS RELIEVING TIPS

1. Eat balanced nutritious diet. No more diet crazes with the pendulum effect.

2. Proper exercise, must take into consideration your present condition. Even deep breathing exercises are stress relieving. Try to walk or swim, exercise your limbs, it is all-beneficial. In water most MS people feel a freedom that is not available on land. Most can propel themselves grace-fully for a few feet at least. It raises self-esteem and accom-plishment levels to an all time high. Meditation should become a daily experience.

I personally swim the length of the pool at least twice. Then I back float two laps, then holding onto the side of the pool I lift my legs—one at a time for a count of fifty…to one hundred, (I had to work up to this one). Then still holding onto the side of the pool I kick to a count of 100, or more if I'm not too tired. Then I swim two more laps if possible. I never exercise to the point of exhaustion, only until I feel tired. If I can't swim I walk a half-mile at least, further if there is time and weather conditions are favorable.

3. Seek out an impersonal support group. This can either be a therapist, an MS chapter support group, or a neighbor:

NOTE: a family member tends to be too close to aid the individual with the chronic disease, no matter how well-meaning and self-sacrificing they are, they may not be able to deal with the added responsibility. Also, by doing this you may be creating a co-dependent in your loved one and you may need to talk with a professional to determine this before accepting the help of your loved one.

4. Build your self-esteem by doing something you know you are good at, that won't burn your energy away. I write, not only because it comes easily to me, but also by writing I find myself understanding my ups and downs in a non-threatening manner.

5. Keep your life in perspective, and realize there will be some things you will have to let go of, but then substitute something else. A friend of mine substituted mental aerobics for physical aerobics. She now is considered a mathematical wizard. So what, that you once jogged ten miles, now walk a mile. Once you supervised dozens of people, now supervise yourself.

6. Determine who you are and what you want. Make a postive you!
Remember: the childhood story about the engine that huffed and puffed up the hill saying over and over again, "I think I can, I think I can, I know I can!"

7. Promote a baseline of information for self-assessment ment; update it regularly.

Start with a list of the things you are doing now. Where you live, how you are living. What you eat, your weight, your likes and dislikes in food. Which of these things do you have control over? What would you like to change. This simple list will add much to your own awareness of your lifestyle. Do it now.

Appendix C
Vitamins And Their Qualities

Vitamins and Minerals   Purpose

A   Assists in fighting infections including respiratory infection.
SOURCE: green & yellow vegetables, eggs, organ meats.

B1   Assists in fighting fatigue, depression, & confu sion. Promotes emotional stability.
SOURCE: Whole grains, liver, beans, wheat germ, brewer's yeast, green vegetables.

B2   Assists in fighting apprehension and insomnia.
SOURCE: Yeast, organ meats, fish, nuts, wheat germ, soybeans.

B3   Pantothenic Acid Asists in converting fat sugar to energy.
SOURCE: Liver, kidney, brewers yeast, sunflower seeds, peanuts

Protein   Assists in forming tissue.
SOURCE: Pork, beef, lamb, veal, fish, chicken, turkey, cheese, nuts, beans, peas.

B6   Aids in the metabolism of fat, assists in fighting nausea and dizziness.
SOURCE: Organ meats, whole grains, walnuts, peanuts, wheat germ, bananas, fish, sunflower seeds.

B12   Necessary for the proper functioning of the immune system and the nervous system.
SOURCE: Yeast, liver, wheatgerm, milk, eggs.

C   Assists in repairing tissue and fighting infections.
SOURCE: Citrus fruits, green pepper, chili, broccoli, spinach, tomatoes, baked potatoes, strawberries.

Potassium   Assists in fighting fatigue and in forming healthy heart muscle
SOURCES: Vegetables, egg, Lecithin.

Calcium   Assists in forming and strengthening bones and acts as a natural sedative.
SOURCES: Milk, bone meal

Magnesium   Acts as a natural tranquilizer and assists in fighting irritability.
SOURCES: Vitamin D, Milk

SOYA LECITHIN SOFTGELS   Found in all cells of the body acts as a emulsifier of fats and aids the nervous system by relaying messages, lowering high blood pressure, etc.

SOURCE: CAPSULES SOFT GELS
(I take 4 a day—every day)

LESS STRESS FAST FOODS

BANANAS (A, B1, B6, C, POTASSIUM)
ALMONDS (B COMPLEX, COPPER, IRON, CALCIUM, PHOSPHORUS)

RAISINS (B1, B6, CALCIUM, POTASSIUM, COPPER)

BROCCOLI (C)

SPINACH (A, MAGNESIUM) WHEAT GERM (B COMPLEX)

SUNFLOWER SEEDS (E, PANTOTHENIC ACID)
MILK AND HONEY (CALCIUM—NATURAL SLEEPING TABLET)

BASIC FOOD GROUPS AND RECOMMENDED DIET

A. BREADS, CEREALS, AND OR GRAIN PRODUCTS (WHOLE GRAIN)
SERVING SIZE: 1 PIECE OF BREAD; ½ COOKED PASTA, 3/4 CUP UNSWEETENED CEREAL OR 1/3 C COOKED RICE

B. FRUITS
SERVING SIZE: 1 PIECE OF ½ C CUT UP; 3/4 CUP UNSWEETENED JUICE

C. VEGETABLES
(DARK GREEN, DEEP YELLOW, STARCHY, OTHERS)
    SERVING SIZE: ½ CUP COOKED OR 1 CUP RAW

D. PROTEIN
LEAN MEATS, EGGS, FISH, POULTRY W/O SKIN, BEANS, NUTS, SEEDS ETC.
    SERVING SIZE: 1 OZ MEAT, FISH, OR POULTRY, 1/4 C BEANS.

E. MILK, CHEESE, YOGURT L/F
SERVING SIZE: 1 C MILK, 1 C YOGURT, 1.5 OZ CHEESE

F. FATS, SWEETS, AND ALCOHOL
SERVING SIZE: ALWAYS REMEMBER MODERATION!

G. THE ABOVE SUGGESTIONS ARE FOR MAINTAIN-ING YOUR CURRENT

WEIGHT. TO DROP WEIGHT EITHER INCREASE ACTIVITY OR DECREASE

FOOD INTAKE. I WOULD START WITH FAT! IF YOU'RE NOT EATING

THIS WAY NOW AND START YOU'LL PROBABLY LOSE WEIGHT ANYWAY OR

AT LEAST FEEL A WHOLE LOT BETTER!

SUBSTANCES TO AVOID

A. REFINED SUGAR

Has no benefit in the human diet, no vitamins, no minerals, no fiber. It's manmade poison—and can be chemically compared to cocaine, both are psychologically additive, both produce strong physical and emotional ef-fects, both derive from common plant sources.

CHOCOLATE: ALL TYPES—has been found to inhibit neurological functioning.

B. FAT

Anything containing fat should be limited. It is linked to the following diseases. Cancer, increases the severity of diabetes, fibrocystic breast disease, gallstones, high blood pressure, obesity, hearing disorders, Meniere's disease.

C. ALCOHOL—BECOMES SUGAR AND FAT IN OUR BODIES

Is implicated in the following diseases; anemia— encourages the excretion of B vitamins; cancer link, hiathal hernia, high blood pressure, ulcers.

D. CAFFEINE/COFFEE/TEA/SODAS

Caffeine enters all organs and tissues of the body within a few minutes of ingestion. Ninety percent is metabolized and only 10% is excreted unchanged in the urine. Caffeine's effects may be subtle and obscured by the multifaceted nature of many chronic disease states.

Some may be thinking; "Hey, Marilyne everybody drinks coffee, tea, or Cola and eats chocolate…can it really be all that bad? Understanding some of the side effects of caffeine may be all that is needed for individuals with MS to discontinue consuming anything with caffeine. I know that if I had been aware of these side effects of caffeine 15-20 years ago I would have prevented several uncomfortable hospital stays eliminating permanent damage to my neural system.

I will only list only the Central Nervous System effects of caffeine. There are others dealing with the gastrointestinal system, respiratory system, kidneys, bladder, prostate, and thyroid infection. It predisposes women to fibrocystic breast disease. Withdrawal symptoms usually cease after two or three days and can include a) headaches, b) drowsiness c) runny nose and nausea d) cotton mouth e) nervousness and irritability f) trembling with a chill g) insomnia h) even depression and an inability to work effectively. These withdrawal symptoms last up to two weeks or a bit more, depending on the level of addiction.

1. Caffeine's Effect on the Nervous System
In children, it may cause damage to the brain and central nervous system development. A survey revealed pregnant women who consume an average of 193 mg of caffeine a day, or 5 or more cups of coffee a day, cause thousands of birth defects.

Caffeine is a powerful central nervous system stimulant. Large doses may impact motor function, where delicate coordination is required. It increases reaction to sensory stimuli, but the post stimulation results in fatigue, lethargy, and depression. All mental and physi cal stimulation ceases when consuming more than two cups or two cola's in two hours. After two cups, coffee, or caffeine, acts to slow all reaction times and impairs thinking ability.

High doses of caffeine can produce symptoms indistinguishable from anxiety neurosis. Caffeine causes nervousness, irritability, muscle tension, and trembling. It can cause headaches, shaky hands, and even hallucinations. High does 20 cups or 400 mg of caffeine, can cause grand mal seizure, respiratory failure, and death.

Caffeine is the principal cause of "restless leg syndrome". This results in insomnia and an uncomfortable feeling caused by involuntary movement, (jerking) of the legs or hands. It has significant effects on muscle contractions/re-laxing smooth muscles and increasing the contraction of skeletal muscles.

Caffeine may mask mental and physical fatigue. This may be dangerous while driving. It interacts with other drugs and decreases barbital-induced sleeping time. Caffeine is habit forming and addictive.

Both coffee and tea destroy thiamine (vitamin B1) because of their high caffeine content. Any heavy caffeine user is likely to be deficient in B1, which is crucial to mental health and tranquility. Lack of thiamine causes nervous exhaustion, fatigue, loss of appetite, loss of memory, depression, constipation, inability to concentrate, feelings of inadequacy, lethargy and intense drowsiness.

Caffeine has been known to trigger psychosis, through its action on a set of chemicals in the brain called neurotrans mitters. These convey messages across microscopic gaps, called synapses, between nerve cells in the brain and muscles.

What about caffeine-free coffee and soft drinks you may now ask? A chemical used in making decaffeinated coffee, (TCE-tricholoroethylene) has been known to cause liver cancer. The National Cancer Institute also warns against using three possible substitutes for TCE. Replacing a chemical with carcinogenic risk with another chemical of unknown risk may result in a more hazardous alternative. In other words, all the side effects of the chemical used in decaffeinated coffer, tea, etc. are still unknown. Caffeine-free soft drinks and sugar-free soft drinks still have substitutes and chemicals. It is best striving to develop a taste for healthy beverages. Think of how much beverage is consumed during a lifetime! It's the fluid your body used to trigger every chemical reaction and enzyme activity in your body. If a few chemicals in the beverages we drink don't make any difference in how people feel, try putting one percent water in a gas tank and see how well a car runs.

The most obvious question following this lengthy aside on the effects of caffeine drinks and chocolate is "If I can't drink coffee, tea, alcohol, soft drinks, or even eat chocolate what is left for me?"

Fresh spring water is my first answer. Everyone should drink up to 8-10 glasses of water a day to provide the body with needed fluid. After strenuous exercise on a hot day, nothing quenches thirst like water. I place the juice of a fresh lemon in a cup of hot water finding it a good way to start the day and it also helped me loss weight.

Next try carbonated spring water (Perrier) plain, lemon, lime, or orange. It can be purchased at any grocery store. It contains no calories, sugar, or chemicals. It is a good, carbonated, refreshing substitute for cola. Next try sugar-free fruit and vegetable juice. A healthy investment could be a vegetable/fruit juicer to produce fresh juice. Nothing tastes better or is healthier for you than freshly juiced fruits and vegetables. Lastly, most stores have natural cereal beverage to replace coffee that are very pleasant tasting. Some popular ones are Sipp, Caffix, and Pero. I have become quite creative with my beverages and I know you will too once you make the commitment to a life without caffeine.

Beverages	Caffeine mg	Caffeine mg
filter drip coffee 110 Decaff Coffee		2
Percolated Coffee		85
Dark Chocolate		80
Instant Coffee		65
Leaf Tea		40
Milk Chocolate		35
Cola not decaff		25
Cocoa		15

Note: Coffee from South America beans usually contains about half as much be an African coffee beans.

E. SODIUM (salt)
Implicated in the following diseases: high blood pressure, water retention, headaches, ulcers

F. Nutrition-wise food storage and preparation is not a science. Home cooking methods used are largely those that have been handed down from generation to generation and date back to the time when the science of nutrition was unknown. The nutrients in many foods are either destroyed or thrown away before the food reaches the table. If health is to be had from the food we grow and buy, care must be taken in the handling and preparation. Many vitamins are destroyed by oxidation and dissolved in water.

Appendix D—Nutrition

BASIC FOOD GROUPS

The following is a list of the four food groups
The Best Proteins
(Little or no fat)
Shellfish   Fish   Chicken w/o skin   Veal
Very Lean Beef trimmed of all visible fat
Second Best Proteins
Low-fat Cottage Cheese   Skimmed or L/f Milk/Yogurt
Dried Peas and Beans   Lentils
Tofu and other soybean-based foods

Carbohydrates (simple and complex)

Starches

Breads	Crackers/Muffins/Rolls/Bagels	Pasta
Potatoes	Rice	Barley
Kasha	Corn/including tortillas	Cereals
Oatmeal/w/o milk		

Sweets (Glucose is only sugar which will produce immediate increase in insulin)

Candy   Cookies   Pie   Cake
Ice Cream   Jams, Jellies Syrup   Soft Drinks
Chocolate * (see appendix)

Fruit won't activate the insulin as quickly, processing of fructose to glucose takes the body time, even though fructose is the sweetest of the sugars.

Appendix E. Definitions

Acupuncture: The ancient art of healing through the meridian points, identified after therapist takes the pulses to determine the area that needs balancing. Balance the whole systems of life energy.

Amino Acids: The organic compounds forming the basic proteins.

Adipose Tissue: Fat tissue cells.

Basal Metabolism: The energy produced by an individual during physical digestive, and emotional rest; measured directly by heat evolved and indirectly by oxygen consumed and carbon dioxide

Biofeedback: A stress reducing form of therapy using machines or meditation.

Betaseron Therapy: Chemical developed in the late 1980's that has had acceptance by FDA for treating remitting-relapsing MS.

Calorie: The unit by which heat is measured.

Co-polyamar-1 Therapy: Chemical developed in the early 1990's that may aid MS patients with remitting-relapsing MS.

Nutrition: The combination of processes by which the living organism receives and utilizes the materials necessary for the maintenance of its functions and for the growth and renewal of its components.

Nutrients: Any substance useful in nutrition
Glycogen: Storage form of glucose in liver and muscles.

Glycolysis: Breakdown of glycogen.

Order of Metabolism: Carbs/Proteins/Fat

R.D.A.: Recommended Daily Allowance. The amounts of various nutrients recommended by the food and nutrition board of the National Research Council as normally desirable objectives toward which to aim in planning practical diets to cover substantially all individual variations in the requirements of people in normal health.

Spontaneous Remission: Partial or complete disappearance of a condition in the absence of all treatment.

T-cells: Building cells of the body.

Visualization: Use of the imagination to create a positive reality.

Wet Cell: Envisioned by Edgar Cayce, this appliance is a modified battery, which allows for realignment of the individual's magnetic body.

Appendix F:
Bibliography and Suggested Readings

1.   Ailes, Roger, You Are The Message; Getting What You Want By Being What You Are; Doubleday, 1989

2.   Ardell, Donald B.; High Level Wellness: An Alternative to Doctors, Drugs, and Disease Bantum Books, 1979

3.   Atkins, Robert C., M.D.; Multiple Sclerosis: Complementary Approach Succeeds Where Conventional Medicine Fails; Vitamin Cottage Magazine; August 1994

4.   Beattie, Melody, Codependent No More, New York, Harper/Hael don, 1987

5.   Black, Claudia, It Will Never Happen to Me, Denver MAC Publishers, 1982

6.   Bowen, Murray, Healing the Shame that Binds You, Pompano Beach Health Communications Inc. 1986

7.   Caprio, Frank M.D. and Joseph R. Berger, Helping Yourself With Self-Hypnosis; Reward Books, 1974

8.   Cayce, Edgar; The Wet Cell; A.R.E. Clinic—Pathways to Health; Phoenix, AZ

9.   Stern, Jess; Edgar Cayce—The Sleeping Prophet; Doubleday & Co., Inc., 1966

10.   Cerney, J. V.; Acupuncture Without Needles; Parker Publishing Co; 1988

11. Chopra, Deepak, MD. Agless Body, Timeless Mind: The Quantum Alternative To Growing Old. Crown Publishers, Inc. 1993.

12. 10. Clarke Jan Illsley, Self-esteem A Family Affair, Minneapolis, Winston Press 1978

13. Colfin, Annemarie, Food and Healing; Winston Press, 1979

14. Connelly, Dianne M., Ph.D.; Traditional Acupuncture: The Law of the Five Elements, Center For Traditional Acupuncture, Inc. 1975

15. Culligan, Matthew J., and Keith Sedlack, M.D.; How To Avoid Stress Before It Kills You; Gramercy Publishing Co; 1980

16.   Davis; Adelle; Let's Eat Right To Keep Fit and Let's Get Well and Let's Cook It Right; New American Library; 1954

17. Dosey, Larry MD. Meaning & Medicine: A Doctor's Tales of Breakthrough and Healing. Bantam Books. 1991.

18. Fackelmann, Kathy A; Traitorous Lymphocytes; Drug Assaults From Leukemia to MS; Science News; Vol. 145; June 1994

19. Fonda, Jane; Yoga, Exercise Workout; D Vision Entertainment Video; 1993

20. Forward, Susan and Craig Buck, Betrayal Of Innocence; Incest and Its Devastation, New York, Viking Penguin; 1988

21. Forward, Susan, Ph.D., Toxic Parents, Overcoming Their Hurtful Legacy and Reclaiming Your Life; Bantum Books, NY, 1989

22. Fossum Merle A. And Marilyn J. Mason, Facing Shame: Families In Recovery, New York, WW Norton & Co; 1986

23. Gawain, Shakti; Creative Visualization; New World Library, 1970, 1990

24. Giesser, Dr. Barbara Diagnosis: The Whole Story, Inside MS Vol 9 #3,, 1991.

25. Griffin, Moira, Going The Distance; E. P. Dutton; 1990

26. Griggs, Rick; Personal Wellness Crisp Publications, 1989

27. Helpern, Howard, Cutting Loose; An Adult Guide to Coming to Terms With Your Parents; NY, Bantam Books, `1978

28. Herman, Juidith, Father-Daughter Incest, Cambridge Harvard University Press, 1982

29. 27. Hirshberg, Caryle; Spontaneous Remission, The Spectrum of Self-Repair; ICD, vol 9, CM.

30. Hittleman, Richard; Richard Hittleman's Yoga, 28 Day Exercise Plan; Bantam Books; 1973

31. Hausman, Patricia and Judith Benn Hurley, The Sugar Blues; Telltale Signs; The Healing Foods, The Ultimate Authority on the Curative Power of Nutrition 1989

32. Kempree, CH, The Battered Child, Chicago university of Chicago Press 1980

33. Klien and Kroll, Erica Levy and Ken. Enabling Romance: A Guide to Love, Sex, and Relationships for the Disabled. Betheseda, Maryland. Woodbine House, 1995.

34. Lerner, Goldhor Harriet, The Dance Of Anger, Harper and Row, 1985

35. Lechtenberg, Richard M.D. Multiple Sclerosis Fact Book. Philadelphia: F.A. Divis Company, 1995.

36. Maxwell, Katie, Bedside Manners; Baker Book House; and 1989

37. Pursuit Of Hope,

38. McNally, David; Even Eagles Need A Push, Learning To Soar In A Changing World; Transform Press; 1990

39. Masters, Robert Ph.D. and Jean Houston, Ph.D; Listening To The Body, The Psycho physical Way To Health and Awareness, Delta Books, 1978

40. Masters, Robert Ph.D. and Jean Houston, Ph.D; Mind Games, the Guide To Inner Space; Delta Books, 1972

41. Miller, Alice, Prisoners of Childhood, NY Basic Books 1981

42. Newton, Matt and Brenda. Brenda's Story: My Life with Multiple Sclerosis. Mercer, Pensylvania, M&B Newton, Inc. 1993

43. Oliver-Diaz, Philip and Patricia A. O. Gorman, 12 Steps To Self Parenting, Health Communications , Inc 1948

44. Ostrander, Sheila and Lynn with Nancy Ostrander; Superlearning, Delacorete Press and the Confucian Press, New York, 1979.

45. Peale, Norman Vincent; The Power Of Positive Thinking; Spire Books, 1952

46. Pollin, MSW Irene. Taking Charge: Overcoming The Challenges of Long-Term Illness. New York: Times/Random House, 1992.

47. Pelletier, Kenneth R.; Holistic Medicine: From Stress To Health; Delta Book; 1979

48. Rector, Linda N.D., Ph.D. How To Be Your Own Herbal Pharmacist. 1995

49. Reuben, M.D., David; Everything You Always Wanted To Know About Nutrition; 1989

50. Rosner, M.D. Louis J. Multiple Sclerosis: New Hope and Practical Advice for People with MS and Their Families. New York: Fireside, Simon and Schuster, Inc. 1995.

51. Silva, Jose; The Silva Mind Control Method; Pocket Books, 1977

52. Sheehy, Gail; Passages; Predictable Crises of Adult Life; Bantum Books, 1974

53. Siegel, Bernie S., M.D.; Love, Medicine & Miracles; Harper & Row, Publishers, New York; 1986

54. Tannen Ph.D., Deborah; You Just Don't Understand; William Morrow and Co., 1990

55. Taylor, Deborah Seymour; The Wet Cell; Venture Inward; July/August 1993

56. Weissberg, Charles L., Dangerous Secrets: Maladaptive Responses to Stress; NY WW Norton & Co 1983

57. Whitefield, Charles L., Healing The Child Within, Pompano Beach, Health Communications Inc. 1987

58. Witkin, Georgia; Social Readjustment Rating Scale; 1991.

59. Woititz, Janet Geringer, Adult Children of Alcoholics, Pompano Beach Health Communications, Inc., 1983

60. Wolf, John K.; Mastering Multiple Sclerosis, A Guide To Management; Academy Books; 1975

61. Wurtman,Ph.D., Judith J.; Managing Your Mind and Mood Through Food, MIT Research Scientist Research Paper, M.I.T. Chemistry

APPENDIX G: EDGAR CAYCE

The sleeping prophet of the early 1900's was a man of extreme vision and insight[52]. His work is far from over as he has made contact from the other side through mediation with myself and others through the continuing work of the A.R.E. Press in Virginia Beach, Virginia. While using the Cayce Wet Cell appliance in April of 1994 I experienced a compelling need to write in my computer journal. Once I hooked up my laptop computer and reattached myself to the Wet Cell appliance I received the channeled message that appears (in the alternative treatment) section of this book. Page 129

Mr. Cayce has attempted to clarify the mystery of the symptoms that I have displayed during the past 20+/- years. He has given me and my caregivers clear and specific guidelines for seeking out healers from all walks of the medical profession. He has also identified the positive results of using certain medicines and chemicals and electromagnetic tools to stop the progression of my condition. I have continued to receive insights into my condition, in the same manner as the first one, each signed with an E.C.

The originial manner of contact between Mr. Cayce and myself was not expected or imagined by myself. Yet I feel it is highly accurate to my condition and since receiving the original message I have made steady progress by using his

---

52. Stern, Jess; *The Sleeping Prophet*; Doubleday & Co., Inc. 1966

prescription. The Wet Cell is a battery-like device that helps the body to realign the magnetic fields that are out of alignment. It is simple and inexpensive. Contact the Cayce center in Tucson, Arizona for specific ordering information.

A definite message that Mr. Cayce has left with me is, "The one who treats him/herself, has an idiot for a patient, and a fool for a doctor. The wise one who seeks out alternative treatments is more likely to find success by keeping the mind open and the heart pure following the prescription while on a clean spiritual path to the all knowing lord through mediation and prayer."

NOTES

Foot Notes

1. Davis, Adelle; *Let's Eat Right To Keep Fit* and *Let's Get Well* and *Let's Cook It Right*; New American Library, 1954

2. Wolf, John K.; *Mastering Multiple Sclerosis: A Guide To Management*; Academy Books, 1975

3. Multiple Sclerosis Society, National Office; 205 East 42nd St. New York, NY 10017 (212) 986-3240

4. Hirshberg, Caryle: *Spontaneous Remission: The Spectrum of Self-Repair*, 4/1993; Noetic Science Review, Sausalito, California.

5. IRS regulations allow any chronic disease sufferer to deduct the cost of equipment recommended by a physician.

6. Sedlacek, Keith, M.D. *How To Avoid Stress Before It Kills You*; Gramercy Publishing,

7. Witkins, Georgia; *Social Readjustment Rating Scale for Stress in the 1990's*; New York

8. Witkin, Georgia; *Social Readjustment Rating Scale*; 1991

9. Cayce, Edgar; *Wet Cell*; A.R.E. Clinic, Pathways to Health, Phoenix, Az. 1-(602)-955-9206.

10. Cayce, Edgar; Wet Cell Appliance; [528-6) & [261-27]

11. Connelly, Diane M. Ph.D.; *Traditional Acupuncture: The Law of the Five Elements*; Center for Traditional Acupuncture, Inc. 1980

12. Cerney, J.V.; *Acupuncture Without Needles*; Parker Publishing Co., 1988

13. Griggs, Rick; *Personal Wellness*; Crisp Publications, 1989

14. Connelly, Diane M. Ph.D.; *Traditional Acupuncture: The Law of the Five Elements*; Center for Traditional Acupuncture, Inc. 1986

15. Tinker, Mary. MS Chatter, 1995.

16. Hittleman, *Richard; Richard Hittleman's Yoga, 28 Days Exercise Plan*; Bantam Books, 1973

17. Culligan, Matthew J. and Keith Sedlack, M.D.; *How To Avoid Stress Before It Kills You*; Gramercy Publishing Co.; 1980

18. Reuben, David, M.D.; *Everything You Always Wanted To Know About Nutrition; 1989*

19. Davis, Adelle; *Let's Eat Right To Keep Fit and Let's Get Well and Let's Cook It Right*; New American Library; 1954

20. Hausman, Patricia and Judith Bean Hurley; *The Sugar Blues: Telltale Signs: The Healing Foods, The Ultimate Authority on the Curative Power of Nutrition*; 1989

21. *Prevention*; P.O. Box 7585, Red Oak, IA 51591-2585

22. *Longevity*; P.O. Box 3226; Harlan, IA 51593-2406

23. *The Silva Mind Control Method*; Silva, Jose; Pocket Books; 1977

24. *Sick and Tired of Feeling Sick and Tired: Living with Invisible Illness*; Donoghue, Paul J. Ph.D. and Mary E. Siegel, Ph.D.; Norton & Company, New York; 1992

25. *Take Charge of Your Emotional Life: Self-Analysis Day by Day; Langs, Robert, M.D.; Henry Holt and Company; New York; 1991*

26 Wurtman, Judith J. Ph.D. *Managing Your Mind and Mood through Food*. MIT Research Scientist Paper, M.I.T. Chemistry 1990

27. Reuben, David, M.D. *Everything You Always Wanted To Know About Nutrition; 1990*

28. Colfin, Annemarie; *Food and Healing*; Ballentine Books, 1986

29. Wurtman, Judith J. Ph.D. *Managing Your Mind and Mood Through Food, MIT Research Scientist Research Paper*, MIT Chemistry

30. Reuben, David, M.D. *Everything You Always Wanted To Know About Nutrition, 1989*

31. Colfin, Annemarie, *Food and Healing*; Ballentine, 1986

32. Reuben, David, M.D. *Everything You Always Wanted To Know About Nutrition*; 1989

33. Hausman, Patricia and Judith Benn Hurley, *The Sugar Blues: Telltale Sign: The Healing Foods, The Ultimate Authority on the Curative Power of Nutrition*, New York, 1989

34. Gawain, Shakti, *Creative Visualization*; New World Library, San Rafael, CA. 1978

35. Gawain,Shakti; *Creative Visualization*; New World Library, San Rafael, CA, 1978

36. *Creative Visualization: Use the Power of Your Imagination to Create What You Want In Your Life*; Gawain, Shakti; New World Library; San Rafael, California; 1978

37. Tannen, Deborah Ph.D.; *That's Not What I Meant*; Ballentine Books, 1986

38. Tannen, Deborah, *You Just Don't Understand: Women and Men In Conversation*; Ballantine Books; New York, 1990

39. Tannen, Deborah, Ph.D. *You Just Don't Understand*, William Morrow and Co. New

40. Pelletier, Kenneth R.; *Holistic Medicine*; Delta Book; 1979

41. Beatty, Melody; *Co-Dependent No More*; Doubleday, 1989

42. Masters, Robert Ph.D. & Jean Houston, Ph.D.; *Mind Games, The Guide To Inner Space*; Delta Books, 1972

43. Alies, Roger; *You are the Message: Getting What You Want By Being What You Are*; Doubleday, 1989

44. Masters, Robert Ph.D. & Jean Houston Ph.D.; *Listening To The Body, The Psycho physical Way To Health and Awareness*; Delta Books, 1978

45. Sheehy, Gail; *Passages; Predictable Crises of Adult Life*, Bantam Books, New York, 1976

46. Tannen, Deborah; *You Just Don't Understand*; Ballantine Books, New York, NY, 1990

47. Siegel, Bernie S., M.D.; *Love Medicine & Miracles: Lessons Learned About Self-Healing from a Surgeon's Experience with Exceptional Patients*; Harper & Row Publishers, New York; 1986

48. Atkins, Robert C., Dr.; Multiple Sclerosis; Complimentary Approach Succeeds Where Conventional Medicine Fails; Vitamin Cottage Health Hotline; August 1994.

49. Koehler Company, P.O. Box 1508, Mt. Vernon, Washington, 98278; Phone 206-424-6025 or Fax (206) N424-6029

50. Jamison, Kaleel; *The Nibble Theory, and the Kernel of Power*; Paulist Press, New York, 1984

51. McNally, David; *Evan Eagles Need A Push: Learning To Soar In A Changing World*; Transform Press; 1990

52. Stern, Jess; *The Sleeping Prophet*; Doubleday & Co., Inc. 1966

GLOSSARY DEFINITIONS H

Acupuncture: The ancient art of healing through the meridian points, identified after therapist takes the pulses to determine the area that needs balancing. Balance the whole systems of life energy.

Amino Acids: The organic compounds forming the basic proteins.

Adipose Tissue: Fat tissue cells.

Basal Metabolism: The energy produced by an individual during physical digestive, and emotional rest; measured directly by heat evolved and indirectly by oxygen consumed and carbon dioxide

Biofeedback: A stress reducing form of therapy using machines or meditation.

Betaseron Therapy: Chemical developed in the late 1980's that has had acceptance by FDA for treating remitting-relapsing MS.

Calorie: The unit by which heat is measured.

Co-polyamar-1 Therapy: Or CoPaxone, chemical developed in the early 1990's that may aid MS patients with remitting-relapsing MS

Glycogen: Storage form of glucose in liver and muscles.

Glycolysis: Breakdown of glycogen.

Nutrition: The combination of processes by which the living organism receives and utilizes the materials necessary for the maintenance of its functions and for the growth and renewal of its components.

Novantrone: IV dispenced meedication by MD for progressive MS.

Nutrients: Any substance useful in nutrition

Order of Metabolism: Carbs/Proteins/Fat

R.D.A.: Recommended Daily Allowance. The amounts of various nutrients recommended by the food and nutrition board of the National Research Council as normally desirable objectives toward which to aim in planning practical diets to cover substantially all individual variations in the requirements of people in normal health.

Royal   Rife—Electrometronic   Model   D—BioActive Instrument: The frequency channel are determine by the condition one is treating for. This amazing tool helps realign the body to ultimate health. By following the instructions closely any dis-ease identified may achieve remission with the condition. Long term use is suggested for overall stability.

Spontaneous Remission: Partial or complete disappear-ance of a condition in the absence of all treatment.

T-cells: Building cells of the body.

Visualization: Use of the imagination to create a positive reality.

Wet Cell: Envisioned by Edgar Cayce, the Sleeping Profit in the 1930's, this appliance is a modified battery which allows for realignment of the individual's magnetic body.

EPILOGUE

Courage and tenicity make strange bedfellows,
and they each teach powerful lessons.

M. V. Mabery 1994

ABOUT THE AUTHOR

Marilyne is a prolific writer of fiction and non-fiction. Her interests are as varied as the Encylopida Bricanna. This diary is just the tip of the iceberg to her published efforts. The following modified material in the form of a self-help diary is offered as a testment to what an open mind can achieve.

INDEX

0-595-20840-1

www.ingramcontent.com/pod-product-compliance
Lightning Source LLC
Chambersburg PA
CBHW061407280526
45784CB00001B/397